For my wife, Mercye
and children,
Jason, Jacqui, Krista, Meggan and Katie

Thank you so much! God bless!

Gary

Introduction

This is a true story, my story. To protect the innocent friends and my students, situations described will be very real without mentioning specific names involved. There have been people very dear to me that I may have unintentionally hurt or disappointed due to my handicapping condition, mental illness, or even sinful behavior. For this reason, I will leave names out of this book. I will stick to the topic of being "Special Education" and never really properly diagnosed until later in life and spending over twenty years teaching Special Education students with some of the same kind of problems as I.

1

Breakdown!

It started right before my senior year of high school, the week before to be exact. Now, my classmates may have observed something wrong with me, the way I was behaving during the preceding spring semester. My mom had mentioned it without any specifics.

I had been with the same classmates since kindergarten, so we knew each other quite well. We had been raised near a very rich oil field, a national forest, cattle, ranches, and farms in northern Santa Barbara County. It was a great place to grow up! The week before school started, one of my best friends and I attended a district church camp meeting California. There were a variety of fun and inspirational activities for high school-aged youth on a Christian college campus. Personally, I wouldn't miss this experience right before school started!

I had already put upon myself some pressures and high expectations. I wanted to be a better trumpet player and a better football player, as well as to finish preparing myself for college. So, if I felt pressure going into my senior year, it was mostly self-imposed. I am mentioning this, because maybe, it had a lot to do with what was about to happen! Back to Camp Meeting, it was so important to me right before school got started, because of the inspiration I received. It gave me a 'shot-in the-arm' to have a better year at school and deepen my faith in my Creator. It was important because of being raised in a God-fearing home; I chose to adopt the faith of my father and my grandfather as mine whole-heartedly!

The year was 1964, mental illness was not mentioned in those days. It was not understood, that's for sure. I suppose it was something to be rather ashamed to admit, should it be in your family. How could it ever happen to a fine, upstanding Christian family anyway? If a family was with mental illness back in those days, it must be a judgment passed down to parents from God for not being good or responsible. Whose fault was it that this was happening? Shameful guilt and exasperation on the part of parents that didn't know what to think or do! This describes a little bit what it was like back then to consider that there was such a thing called mental illness, even though those words wouldn't have been used. People would have jumped ahead to throwing around descriptive words like crazy or insane knowing there were institutions for people like that. It was a scary subject at best; especially for parents.

Every Labor Day in my hometown, high school football players made their way to our school to check out football pads, helmets, and uniforms to be ready for the first day of school. In 1964, I did not make it back home for Labor Day. I had spent the summer making sure I was well conditioned for my senior year of football. I did my best to keep up with my best friend to be ready to play alongside him as running back for the Bears, to defend our championship.

We were at Camp Meeting where my heart and mind had been burdened for my classmates back home and their spirituality or lack of it. Some negative thoughts crept into my heart and mind attempting to make me believe I was a failure at sharing my faith with my classmates. At some time in the middle of the week, I had a turning point and started believing the opposite. It was like a dark room in which windows are opened to the glorious entrance of warm streaming sunlight. The negative thoughts had been lying when the truth had been revealed to show I had done my best, and just needed to continue doing my best and not fret about it.

Then my mind took off with a euphoric response. I imagined my classmates becoming more spiritual and praying toward that end.

I started losing sleep and getting more and more hyper. My nervous system was really hyped up! If people talked to me they (understand-ably) did not understand my response. I must have sounded con-fused. It did not make sense. It did not relate to the here and now. A by-stander would think I was high on drugs.

I was going through my first bi-polar euphoric episode. The term 'bi-polar' had most likely not been invented yet. Most people only think of severe depression in relation to bi-polar. Through most of my life, my episodes were euphoric instead. My mind did not really play tricks on me, but my imagination took me a little more than an arm's length out of touch with reality.

This book is not about my religious experiences as much as it is about my own personal struggles with emotionally handicapping conditions. Later on, it was the teaching of students with emotional disturbance.

In the middle of the week before Labor Day, it was brought to my parents' attention that something was wrong with me. After they checked me out for themselves, I found myself on my way to the hospital, near my grandfather's house. I remember being able to look out the window of my hospital room at night and see the lights of the Ferris wheel at the Valley Fair. It must have been really scary for my parents; they had no clue what was wrong. Instead of going home, soon I was transported to a county hospital's psychiatric wing.

At some point, my parents believed that their son was having a 'nervous breakdown.' I was in a ward with adults and I wasn't quite seventeen yet. A 'breakdown' seemed to not be as abrasive as the term 'mentally ill.' I am sure it was hard for them to not feel guilt, like they had done something wrong; when actually they were wonderfully supportive parents, in every aspect of life.

Techniques for dealing with emotional disturbance back then were a world away from present practices, and distanced (or advanced) by forty-eight years. For the most part, the hospital staff was kind and caring. The other patients were middle aged and older, they also were friendly and very interesting people to meet. I met a couple patients that had been in the Olympics, a grocery chain exec-utive; and a Professor of Spanish writing a textbook.

There was an experience that was hard for me, in the process of trying to adjust to medications; and I suppose, while the doctor was deciding what would be of best benefit to me. There was a medicine that worked fairly well if accompanied by another. The medicine back then was called Stelazine, but had to have Cogentin with it. Until they figured that out, I would have uncontrollable muscle spasms. They treated me like I could control my spasms with my will! That was upsetting to me! They would put me on a gurney and strap me down! They would give a shot and sedate me with a shot of 50 mg of Mellaril, which would put me to sleep.

I liked occupational therapy time which included a variety of crafts. Working with hands was enjoyable and therapeutic. Come to think of it, it was a measurement of the health of one's nerves. If I were a patient with a project and couldn't focus, I could feel that my nerves were still not right and not healthy yet.

As I was an impressionable teenage boy, I liked a rather pretty, California-sun-tanned nurse. She took time to advance my skills at ping pong. It was one of those special times she made just for me. Being an athlete and competitor, I improved as much as I could while I was there, thanks to this special nurse whom no one could defeat at ping pong.

Some medicine I took made me slow, sluggish, and almost lethargic. It caused me to lie around and not activate my mind or body. Somehow, my doctor had to find a 'happy medium' in regard to my meds—sedated but not observable. In retrospect, the terms 'nervous breakdown' could have been easier for my parents to accept, but would not have been too far from the truth. What I learned about 'bi-polar' many years later could make some sense of my first 'breakdown.' Bi-Polar—one type meant a chemical (like an electrolyte) was missing in my body to connect the endings of nerves. At the time, I would have had a different diagnosis that was a misdiagnosis; which makes more sense now about the unraveling of my nerves. Because I was under age in an adult hospital ward, I don't know what kind of struggles my doctors went through with me to know when I was really ready to go home.

It is hard to imagine being in the hospital for ten weeks. That's how long I was there. I was allowed weekend passes at some point. These gave me a feel for what my nerves could handle or not.

Probably about halfway through my stay at the hospital, I was allowed to go home for the Homecoming game at my high school. My emotions were charged! Football is an emotional game. I had wanted to be playing in that game! I was very excited to be home where my lifetime friends were—my classmates! That was a very different kind of emotion.

Cold weather sets your nerves on edge to some extent. It was cold. A mix of complex feelings and excitement overloaded my nerves. I couldn't bring myself to even stay for the end of my senior year's Homecoming Game to see if we won! It really hit me how sick I was or how sick I'd been! My nervous system couldn't handle so much excitement! I wasn't ready to be home!

Talking about an overload on my nerves and an inability to handle pressure is rather ironic in a way, because I chose a life of pressures, and staying calm under pressure. Let me explain, I chose to be an athlete, expecting to need an athletic scholarship to afford to go to college. Contributing to the success of a championship basketball team required staying cool and calm in adversity.

My junior year in high school, I wrote my own competition arrangement piece for competing in a talent contest. It was concert variations on a gospel song for trumpet. It put me in the finals over the LA area against two fine pianists. Nowadays, it is not fair for a single note instrument to compete against pianists. At the time, it was very intense and stressful, competing with professional type techniques on trumpet!

At school, my friend and I took turns playing the highest notes for trumpets in the school band. The competition was keen between us. In all these scenarios, the ability to handle pressure calmly was required. Consciously, I didn't think about it. I loved playing sports and I loved playing my trumpet. Being calm came from confidence developed over a period of years. Could all these moments under stress be piled and working against my nervous system and adding to the breakdown?

I don't really know that answer; but it makes me wonder. I did not return to school until the second semester. Even though I missed the first semester of my senior year, I had enough units toward graduation to only need two classes in summer school to graduate.

I was back in school with medications to help my nerves stay balanced. Because I missed my senior year of football, my coach wanted me to come back in the fall to play fullback for the Bears and then graduate the following January. This presented a dilemma because part of me wanted to be done and start college in the fall of 1965. Part of me wanted to earn a football scholarship the 'old fashioned' way—with hard work (before I leave). My classmates and I had been in school together for over twelve years. It was touching to know they were upset when I wasn't allowed to walk through the graduation ceremony with them.

2

College Bound!

I decided to go to community college in the fall. If I still needed an athletic scholarship, I would earn it there. In those days, I was ineligible to play ball the first year out of my home community college district. I weight lifted with a football coach all year (for P.E.) and practiced with the baseball team even though I didn't get to play. It was called 'red-shirting.'

Majoring in music in college seemed natural because it was a strength of mine. It seems like my first year of college went very well and I pulled over a B average including a 'D' in Philosophy. Eighteen years old and was lost when the professor asked me to write a paper, philosophizing about something. Well I didn't. My grade took a nose dive. I didn't know to go see the professor and get him to explain what he wanted.

I finished my year 'red-shirting' on the baseball team and performing in the college Theatre Dept. production of *The Music Man*. I was in the barbershop quartet singing the high tenor part. That production was one of the most fun experiences of my life!

How did my nerves stay in 'tact' for a whole year? We had to remind ourselves that my medicine was only a temporary 'fix,' not permanent. It brings up the question how long will it last? And what then?

I have a theory about how I was able to 'last' my whole freshman year without problems. I honestly thought that vigorous weight lifting for football helped keep my nerves healthy. I later had met a minister that had gone through a 'nervous breakdown' and learned that vigorous exercise kept him healthy and able to handle pressures of being a minister. So, I think my theory may be good to some degree.

By the end of my first year, I was in great shape and very strong. For versatility, I shot baskets with the basketball team during the summer, and they thought I could make that team as well.

A family vacation took us to Iowa and South Dakota to see my grandmother and bring back a horse to California for my little brother. I talked to the football Coaches of Dakota Wesleyan University. They showed interest in me and wanted me to come back to California and play community college football and transfer to DWU.

In the last 'minute,' I decided not to play football so I would focus on other sports. The basketball coach wouldn't take me. I honestly thought he was trying to pull a 'power' play on me to get me out on the football field. I'm sure he knew I was one of the four strongest men in the school, but I had made up my mind.

I suddenly stopped all vigorous exercise and easily started gaining weight until I had gained about thirty pounds. Emotionally, I had somewhat an up and down start to my second year of college. By putting on weight, I wasn't as healthy overall, during my second year.

The changes weren't finished. As the second semester started I was set on being third baseman on the baseball team. My coach was going to run-off my extra thirty pounds. Then I was really worried about my Biology grade. It was a late night class, and I had to be in the music dept. early in the morning every day.

All afternoon, I belonged to the baseball team. I decided to avoid a bad grade in Biology by dropping the class. This meant I also had to drop baseball because I didn't carry enough units to continue playing.

Wow! I could have easily been playing football, basketball, and baseball at community college level! Then I wasn't playing anything at all except trumpet. It had taken me a year of hard work, but I became soloist in the Symphonic Band and Pep Band, in which I was playing Herb Alpert music at football and basketball games.

If I was in anyway stressed about not earning an athletic scholarship, I had a big surprise coming!

Before that happened, I had my first relapse during college. Luckily, I got to use my Spring Break to pull myself and my nerves back together, not having to miss any school for my emotional handicap. I had to focus on being a music major. My best subjects were music theory and composition, as well as the hard work that went into being the top trumpet player.

My big surprise came at the end of the school year. My father's employer, ARCO oil company, offered me a scholarship to continue my music education wherever I wanted to transfer. What am I saying? I suddenly did not need an athletic scholarship at all! I had an oil company scholarship! My setbacks emotionally, about not playing ball and needing a scholarship seemed to all be redeemed by this new scholarship.

I gave myself a chance by my progress as a musician and the advancement of my skills as a young composer. So I had just earned my scholarship with academics and talent. This is thanks to the oil company merger that formed Atlantic Richfield Company that afforded opportunities for Scholarships.

Everything seemed to be working out to transfer to a four-year school and work on a Bachelor's degree in Music. I had taken a year and a half to have a relapse with my nerves; but this time it wasn't a whole lot more than a bump in the road. I had survived two years of college and things were looking up.

My overweight worked off in the hot summer sun of ARCO oilfields. My scholarship covered whatever money I did not make during the summer following the college school year.

3

College Transfer

My choice for a school was a small Christian college with a fairly good music department. It had turned out some excellent secondary music teachers for big public schools. Going there was something I had looked forward to since I was young.

My choice in schools dates back to inspiration as early as junior high school when I heard musical performances by representatives of the school. On the back burner of my mind was the fact that my parents went to a church college that was part of the denominational system in which I had just enrolled. They were happy about the education they were receiving at the outbreak of WWII and had to quit. Another artistic dilemma I found myself in, to do with the part of me that is a composer. This school that has the most qualified professors did not have time for young composers. It was important, if possible, to find a channel for my talents at least.

I must say, the college did 'pick-up' on this before I got started. I entered the college as a transfer student more advanced in music theory and composition than the Bachelor's degree graduates. I was called to the Vice President's Office. He sat down quite concerned about my advanced skill in composition. He shared with me he was aware of grades and gifts in the area of music theory.

What he said to me next 'blew-me-away!' He said I could go to the number 1 music school in the country—Indiana University. If not, I could go to a top Music Composition school—University of Southern California. He reminded me that my scholarship would be good anywhere I went. It wasn't for a definite amount, it was based on need. He didn't want to see my gifts as a composer getting squelched in a Christian school that didn't have time to help me develop them.

Considering my present perspective on the topic, it was quite amazing that a university officer could be so sensitive! Why is this an important part of my story? Two reasons— one is that I chose to stay; which set me up to be frustrated artistically; second, has to do with famous composers that you may have heard might have been bi-polar or suffered from mental health problems. Of course, I'm not a famous composer, but I do have mental health issues that had not been completely resolved or properly diagnosed, and a passion for music composition.

Through classes offered, I did learn somehow orchestration and arranging skills. Composition development was on hold. The greatest value musically in this small college was performance experiences—concert choir, voice lessons, chamber singers, concert band and oratorio orchestra. These experiences were invaluable as a base of musical knowledge that would be useful to a composer.

Transferring to this school took some adjusting. The pressure was off to need to be an athlete of any kind. I guess if I decided to participate in intercollegiate sports, it would be for the recreation of it.

During the years before my transfer, I had studied what was happening in the area of basketball. 'In house' was one of the greatest teams in the history of the school! This year's basketball team had a First Team All-American who was also a National Indoor High Jump Champ, thus an All-American in two sports.

Well, I decided to try out for this team. I would be happy to be the last man on the bench, because I knew this team was going to Kansas City to play in the Nationals of the NAIA! I tried out. I stood at only five foot eleven. The team was very kind, and started teaching me how to 'dunk' a basketball. They showed me how to approach the basket due to my lack of height. I was two hundred pounds, but had very strong legs. I had above average ball-handling skills and good 'outside' shooting skills.

Then came the day I had to sit down and have a talk with the head coach. He said that I was a football quarterback but I wasn't learning his system fast enough. He was going to have to cut me from the team. He said my ball-handling skills and shooting skills were excellent. He thought I could play high-level intramural ball, learn to work systems and come back next year and not just make the team but as high as six-man on the team. The number six man is the first man to be substituted into the game of basketball. This is how I was cut from a team for the first time in my life!

The team became as good as everyone expected. When they went to Kansas City to the Nationals, they got beat by 3rd ranked team in the country by 1 point.

I did play in the high level intramural league and averaged fifteen points a game. When it came down to it, I missed going to Kansas City. That took the wind out of my college basketball sails.

I don't know how many people know about this. The wrestling coach approached me, knowing I had played football in high school. He had a position for me on the wrestling team at the weight class, 190lbs. He could field a team for dual matches without a member at 190. This was how he expressed that he had a special spot just for me.

I didn't know what to think. My parents came from the Midwest where wrestling was much bigger than on the West Coast. I had cousins that were on high school wrestling teams and great-uncles that were semi-pro wrestlers, knowing all that made it harder to just say no without thinking about it. I needed to have a doctor when I was sixteen years old, and told that he may not want to release me with his blessing to participate in college wrestling. The problem with bringing this up now, is that, it requires a story in explanation.

When I was sixteen, I was on the first championship Varsity Football Team in the history of our high school. My best skills that I had to offer were at quarterback and fullback. For the first time in my life, I was sitting on the bench because the starting backs were veterans.

They had already spent a whole season at their positions. The fullback was destined to be a Pro-Fullback with the Los Angeles Rams, so he was almost impossible for opponents to stop. I had been his 'understudy' on the junior varsity football team as sophomore the year before, until I broke my ankle.

I was on the verge of scoring every time I touched the ball during practice. My coach started designing plays just for me. We tried them 'out' against the varsity and they broke my ankle. I only brought it up to say that, as a junior, making back-up quarterback was the best I could do. I had a psychological block to get over before I could start carrying the ball again as a fullback (due to my ankle break).

I remember the coach sending me into a game to quarterback the 'starting' running backs to see how we got along, I guess. We moved down the field fairly quickly because our running backs could not be stopped. I just had to get them the ball. When we were getting close enough to score, it was in the plans for me to throw my first varsity touchdown pass. No one knew I had promised my first touchdown pass to one particular teammate. I dropped back to throw and one of my friends was all by himself over to the right and ready to make a touchdown. The one I promised the ball to was under the goal posts surrounded by three Eagles. I threw a bullet right down the middle! He had to wrestle to keep them from taking the ball from him; but there was no way he wasn't coming down without the ball! Now I need to work my way toward why this relates to whether I wrestle on the college team or not. As you may remember, we were raised in an ARCO oil town. It did not happen too often, but we did make it to a rival oil town, Chevron (Standard Oil), for the purpose of matching up in sports in some way, even though their town was ten times larger than ours.

In *their* local newspaper they had a full page article on our football team—the best in school history. Now their high school had just fielded one of the greatest football teams in their school history! I believe that this was fuel enough for the small riot we were about to have between oil town rivals!

Football season was over. There were pre-season basketball games scheduled between us, because their school was so much bigger they put their J.V. team against our Varsity. Before that game, our J.V. team would play their 'B' team.

I am sure it was coincidence, but these were basketball games between our two great football teams! I was the Captain of the JV Team from my school in the first game. After the game, my teammates and I were so hungry we walked down to get a hamburger before we went back to watch the next game. At least that was our plan.

Guys from the other school started following us. We didn't know what they were doing. Suddenly, a guy ran up beside me! I turned my head to see what was up, and knocked me 'out' cold. My size at that time was about five foot ten and 175 pounds. A few months later, I was told the guy that hit me was a 225-pound All-Conference lineman from their great football team. I never remembered really waking up from the evening until we were on the bus and on the way home. I remember being in a daze and hearing that they had tried to run over some of us with cars before we got out of town. There were rival oil companies and great athletic teams, but underneath all that, I'm told that certain farm boys on our teams were absolutely hated and their lives were in danger whenever they came to this town. I guess that I looked like one of those guys from the back. So it wasn't because I was on the football team or captain of the basketball team that had just played, it was mistaken identity. They thought I was one of their most hated. I do remember policemen coming to our school the next week, trying to sort out what happened and who did what. This little ARCO/Chevron riot led me to the chiropractor. I had some vertebrates out of place in my neck. The impact of the blow was so great that the curvature of my neck eventually was reversed!

My doctor thought that college wrestling would be the worst thing I could do for my neck. I do remember being a part of initiating incoming freshmen with a variety of games and competitions. We were up for an all night walkathon and I wrestled the heavy weight wrestling champ from Hawaii. God was our audience in the middle of the night. He pinned me once, quickly. Then he couldn't do it again because of my quickness. We became friends and music majors together. Wrestling made it a little harder to make a decision for the coach. The doctor's warning won out though; and that is why I walked away from the opportunity to be on the wrestling team.

About every fifteen to eighteen months, I would have a relapse. My nerves would need a 'break' from the stresses of college life. As my disappointments piled up and other college related frustrations added in, my grade average went down and I lost my oil company scholarship. Some of my feelings included wishing I could only study music and not have to study biology, physics, and all the other subjects needed for a Bachelor of Arts degree.

My bipolar episodes included losing touch with reality, unraveling nerves, and straining relationships. It usually required me to leave school for a few days with my parents. My psychiatrist was a good ways out of town in Santa Barbara. At some point, my doctor came to the conclusion that my problems were not psychological. He decided that the basis of my problems were chemical. Like some kind of "chemical imbalance." He was really on the right track, and this was before the age of bipolar.

It was kind of amazing, because my doctor was so close to a real solution. At some point during a break from school, my doctor had me come to Cottage Hospital in Santa Barbara to try some new medicine. It was Lithium. This was a natural substance that was already in the body. He would keep me in the hospital long enough to get the substance elevated to a therapeutic level.

In retrospect, Lithium has become a major solution for bipolar. My doctor was really close to discovering it. I am sure what determined—clinically—a therapeutic level had not been established. Lithium was never quite the right stuff for me personally. It seemed to slow me down too much. It didn't make me lethargic, but almost.

Somewhere around my junior year, my grades were running lower and lower setting me up to lose my scholarship. Keep in mind I took two years to be a sophomore and was on a track to not finish until my fifth year, only because I was a little low on units upon transferring in, to be considered a Junior.

I got a letter from the head football coach at Dakota Wesleyan University wanting me to come back to South Dakota and play quarterback on their football team. I had some skills I started developing as a junior in high school, partly inspired by watching Steve Spurrier play for the University of Florida. I could take the ball, run out to the right, and throw it on the 'run.' I taught myself to run to the left and throw on the run—the hardest throw for a right-hander to make. I learned to make these throws in the backyard at home with the help of my mom's giant lilac bush. It would catch the ball every time. I also taught myself to throw a 'jump' pass. I would jump straight up in the air and throw a short and extremely accurate pass. I had also been an understudy to a pro running back in high school, making my skills difficult to defend on the gridiron.

The town where this college was located was also where my uncle lived. My uncle was known there as a professional horse trainer. I was hoping to be able to stay with my uncle if I went back to play college football. He had two boys a little older than me that probably left the house kind of empty when they joined the Army and Navy. My cousins did leave a couple little sisters behind. I am sure had I gone, my uncle would be happy to have me around to help haul hay and put up hay for his friends. He would have had me working hard for room and board and been proud if his nephew made quarterback of the DWU Tigers. He, himself, played football in the US Army.

After all this hoopla, I decided not to go in retrospect, I hate to think if I might have gotten sick when my eighteen-month 'hour glass' ran out and I was if staying with my uncle. I wouldn't have wanted to put that on him. Going was a happy thought. Few people knew about this opportunity. I had wanted to play college football since age twelve. Another old dream of mine laid to rest, because of mainly my mental health handicap.

As I developed a friendship with a girl in my junior and senior year, it only added a complexity of emotions to my mental health handicap, and the struggles and disappointments of my college experience. At some point, our relationship became unhealthy in the name of helping my nerves. We were engaged at the same time that I was less and less successful with my grades; which gave less and less hope of getting into graduate school. In turn, the future seemed more dismal for me, let alone to think about bringing someone with me. I am so glad my engagement didn't last much longer than two or three months, because I was in a downward spin toward a crash landing! She cared too much to put her through what was coming next.

In the midst of everything going on my senior year of school, I found myself for the first time in my life not being able to compete in athletics because of low grades. When I was a junior, the track team was rebuilding and recruited me to learn to throw a discus and later javelin and shot put.

After the second quarter of school my senior year, right before the track and field season started, I pulled a report card that was below a 'C' average. That stopped my participation on the track team. One of my grades went down because of failing to take the final exam. A decent grade on the final would have saved my track season.

I found myself surrounded by three black men in a local donut shop. I was cornered until they had their say with me. They were from the track team. They were each about to break the school record in their respective events, 100m, 200m and 800m sprints. They told me that they were all good at what they did; but that I was the only one on the team that potentially should be going to the nationals with the discus. In practice, I did only half of a spin and was within two feet of the school record. Normally, fifteen feet can be added to that kind of throw to estimate my potential. That is why these teammates were there to encourage me to not give up. The professor was involved, he said he would change my grade if I would take the final and do a satisfactory job on it.

My nerves were about to come unraveled under the stress of everything else, so I never got back to that final or my potential to be an All-American in track and field. My throw was not a far enough distance to compete for a major university, but it was very good for a small Christian college. There were some interesting stories about pulling low grades in music. When it came to doing final projects in Choral Arranging or Orchestration (music writing), we had to copy it in ink (a pen, something like calligraphy) on to music manuscript paper. This was before Wite-out, Xerox copiers, or computers with music writing programs. If we made a mistake, there was only one way to correct it. We had to take an old fashioned razor blade and scrape off any mistake. It was so tedious, especially for someone a little messy like me. I was late getting my projects turned in. Every day that I was late, my grade went down. So, I may have received a 'D' on the project but the quality of my work was 'A.' That was really frustrating and demotivating. At that level, it was also disheartening because I wanted to be a music theory professor someday. I did not know how I was going to get into graduate school if my grades kept going down. I was projected to graduate in 1970.

4

Missing Graduation Again

It was a bit of a commute, but as I got closer to graduation, I began staying with my second cousin and her family. Her husband was a graduate of my school. The last quarter of school before graduation, my mother made the decision that she wanted me to get a doctor for me close to school to insure my graduation.

This idea was disastrous, at least for the moment; even though it worked out eventually. Let me explain what happened. I transferred to a doctor close to my school as opposed to one in Santa Barbara, so far out of town.

It sounded okay. At least I understood why my mother wanted to do this. When I went in to see this new doctor, he said he wanted me to stop taking all medicine that I was on, and immediately start taking Thorazine. It just so happens I had missed enough classes in each subject that I could not afford to miss any more classes or I would be dropped from them.

My sudden overnight change in meds was very dramatic in its results! It made me so unbelievably paranoid I could not go to school! I was never so paranoid before or since! I could not step out of my cousin's house. That medicine was making me sick, so sick, I could not function, or face anybody! No way could I go anywhere! I was dropped from my classes, and had already rented my graduation gown. Well, graduation was off for me! I was a real mess! I missed graduation again!

Somehow, I ended up at my grandpa's house; which was a great place to 'regroup' and pull myself together. I needed to start my life all over and figure out a new direction to go and 'step out' in that direction. I am sure I renewed my dependence on Stelazine, gladly, and got Thorazine cleared out of my system. As I got comfortable with grandma and grandpa, I had to think in the direction of who could use the talents of 'an almost' college graduate with over four years of college.(Sometimes a music major takes more than four years because of all the extra units required)

While I was in my last college, I studied Voice with the Chairman of the Fine Arts Department. I also sang in his Concert Choir. Of my many hours that I spent with him, he had a suggestion to how I use my talent, and get started teaching. He thought if I got a job in a Christian school teaching music, he believed there was a substantial need for someone to write instrumental music of a religious nature that could be published and shared with similar schools.

This inspired the direction of my thought. Maybe I could get a job like that as an 'almost graduate.' I got a lead on a job in the East Bay across the bay from San Francisco. I packed a few things and went up there for an interview. While I was there, I called a local church of the denomination in which I was raised and told them I was in town for a Christian high school music teaching job.

I trekked back down to Southern California to my grandfather's house. The school wasn't interested in hiring me; but the biggest surprise phone call came from the church I had casually contacted. They were interested in possibly hiring me. They needed someone to direct activities of the youth group (teenagers) and direct choirs of the church.

Just a reminder, this book is not necessarily about religious experiences in my life, but about my educational handicaps and struggles as well as how they led to teaching students of some of the same conditions. Getting this job was an opportunity to get more experience working with teenagers and using musical talents. This became an experience to build on near a large predominantly black community.

I recruited a junior high-aged basketball team that I would have pitted against any junior high church team in the Bay Area.

At this place of opportunity I had a mentor. I spent much time with him learning about counseling teens and their problems, What I learned was very sound psychologically and I have used it down through the years in working with youth.

After the funds that were supporting me ran out, I had a choice. I could stay and keep my position voluntarily; because the owner of a music store offered me a job teaching music lessons in his stores. He would teach me to teach all the instruments I didn't know. This was at least positive. I didn't have to bail out because of a health condition relapse. The job I was doing at the church earned a good reference for a future job. I chose to leave and ended up in the central part of California and gained even more experience working with teens. I was elected Teen Director of a whole area around Fresno, for a church youth organization. Aside from my musical talent, if I were going to spend my whole life working with teenagers or teaching them; every experience was going to add to my skill and my wisdom.

This time I had to 'bail' after a couple years. I started losing touch and slipped into a dream world based on the partial reality of going back to school with a chance at possibly finishing college. I was studying with the Head of the Music Department and was analyzing a difficult to understand (theoretically) piece of French, turn-of-the-twentieth century orchestra music. My mind was telling me that I was discovering something new in musical structure in a complex piece. It was somewhat like a chemist determining properties of an unknown substance and finding an unexpected element.

My bipolar condition raised its head in a euphoric sense. It dramatized my thoughts a little more than an arm's length out of touch with reality. This time the people in my life closest to me put me in the county hospital psych ward. I was released in two weeks and had to leave town. My mental illness had burned all the bridges behind me all by itself.

5

Why Not Romance?

Before I go on, I must mention that this time I had gone to help a minister in the area and direct the youth and music for him. I met and married his daughter. The marriage lasted less than a year. My nerves were too unhealthy for the pressures and responsibilities of marriage. She had put me in the hospital, walked away to never see me again, and served me divorce papers! I never blamed her for giving up because of what I had put her through; she was young, talented, very caring, and I am sure, devastated! She was not prepared to handle all that!

Any other romances I might mention will not have knowing my condition and my hang-ups may have hurt people that I choose to keep nameless.

My parents got used to me coming home after a stay in the hospital. I had worked on farms and ranches in the area where I was raised since I was thirteen years old. This time, I checked around to see if anyone needed a tractor driver. Soon, I found myself in the seat of a tractor about twelve hours a day, helping farmers get caught up with their 'tractor work.' My nerves were in disrepair. Out there, under the blue sky, and bright California sun, with a powerful tractor under me, it seemed to be quite therapeutic for my nerves (that had completely unraveled again). It felt good to be valued and needed at that moment; even if it was as a farm hand. Before long, however, I found myself back at grandpa's house.

It was such a good place to go when I needed a new direction for my life! I worked through the snows of winter; which is unusual for the edge of a California desert. My place of employment was a convalescent hospital. A male on that job site was in demand a lot for lifting heavy patients or quadriplegics. I spent a few months there before I discovered how 'cheap' it would be to go back to school at a new state college in Bakersfield. I could get a job and pay my own way to finish my degree. Luckily, I had a great uncle in that area who offered me a one bedroom apartment with really cheap rent.

Since I had just come out of working at a convalescent hospital I thought I would try to find that kind of work in Bakersfield. I did not want to work more than 20 hours per week. That would be enough to sustain myself and pay my way through school. I needed to carry a full load and give myself plenty of time to study. I would have to do my senior year over plus one quarter. When my advisor studied my transcripts to see what I needed to graduate. I was excited to find out they would not transfer my bad grades in music! Why was that so great? It gave me an opportunity to restore a 'B' average so that I could have reawakened hope about going to graduate school.

The next bit of good news came about my job. I got a job in a convalescent hospital, but I wasn't going to have to do any 'dirty work.' I would be answering the phones on the weekend, and two half days during the week.

6

How Could I Miss Graduation Again?

It seems that my 'episodes' happened an average of every eighteen months or so. I was so excited to be back on track with my education, even if it meant over seven years spent getting a bachelor's degree in Fine Arts-Music. Because I was so highly motivated at this point in my life, I think I took better care of myself. Most of my eating habits were healthier. Therefore, my nerves were healthier as well. At least until the eighteen-month 'hour' glass ran out, I would be pretty good to finish this personal project.

This was a 'brand new' state college with bright young music professors. It was fortunate for me to be there in a small school to be able to spend more quality time with my professors.

I developed new interests and skills. I discovered that I thoroughly enjoyed doing historical research related to music history or the history of musical style. I wrote two major senior level papers, that I was told, would also help me gain entrance to graduate school.

One of my papers was concerned with reconstructing, historically, a Lutheran service in August of 1724 when a certain cantata of JS Bach was performed in Leipzig. I wrote another paper that was more theoretical. This was musical analysis comparing and contrasting musical settings of Buxtehude and JS Bach of the *Magnificat,* otherwise known as Mary's Song.

I was preparing a Senior Recital in Voice including some of the toughest tenor solos from Handel's "Messiah." Right in the middle of this intense preparation, I got 'strep' throat. To a singer, that's a disaster! Doctor's order was, I was not allowed to sing at all! Doing a recital requires getting your whole body in good shape as well as your voice; not unlike an athlete. Only after the doctor's okay could I start singing again. I had to start all over getting my voice in the shape it took to do the tough 'operatic' type stuff I had to sing. Everything turned out okay, just frustrating.

I was all set to graduate again and it was discovered that I needed a few more units in music study. At least this time, I got to go through the graduation ceremony with a cap and gown even though I wouldn't get a diploma yet.

My faculty advisor was a musicologist in Choral literature. He set up a summer research project in Historical Musicology. I spent forty hours a week for about six to eight weeks creating a comprehensive annotated bibliography of everything in the college library that could be used for research in Historical Musicology. This gave me the units I needed to graduate and prepare me even more for graduate school in musicology. Then I was able to get a diploma dated August 15, 1975.

Along with trying to finish school, I had been applying to graduate schools that offer M.A.'s or PhD's in Historical Musicology. Knowing that the most substantial writings in historical musicology in Europe were written in German, I got a peer tutor to help me 'brush up' on my ability to read German.

Somehow, I knew I might be required to read German as part of an entrance exam for graduate school. Sure enough, I did have one entrance exam in Musicology that had a passage in German to translate. I don't think I handled it well enough to create an option.

7

Graduate Studies in Music

It didn't matter, because I made it in the front door of the University of Southern California School of Music to work on a PhD in Musicology. Halfway into the program, after two years, was an MA degree in Music History. Musician friends I had at the time upon the announcement thought I was 'crazy' to even consider all that musicology study. They had an idea how hard it would be!

I was a composer at heart, so why go in this direction at all? I wanted the background to qualify me to teach music history and music theory. These are the tough core courses for every kind of music major and degree.

Rather than cry over 'spilt milk' of professors not having time for young composers, I desired to be a part of the solution. I actually wanted to go back to the school that didn't have time for creativity, as a replacement for a retiring Music History professor. Then, I would make sure I had time to help develop young composers.

Unfortunately, I was nearing the time when the sands of my 'hourglass' was close to running out—my eighteen-month 'hour' glass. I was working as a music teacher and a music director at an inner-city church in South Central LA. This was enough of a job to get me started in graduate school at USC no less. If anything could set off the euphoric end of my bipolar with pure circumstances, it seems like this could do it!

Actually, I didn't believe this was really possible; but I had to be really, really excited about the developments in my life! Barely into this 'dream come true' life, reality started slipping through my fingertips, and my nerves began to unravel. When it got bad enough that I started not making sense in normal conversation, the people closest to me put me into one of the two most serious state mental health hospitals in California, the Metropolitan State Hospital. I only had to be there for two weeks. My new friends didn't know for sure what to do with me as my parents were out of state. I guess they thought if it were, there would be no bill to pay when I got out. After all these years, I only remember one traumatic experience while I was there. I am sure at first that they gave me high doses of Mellaril. This knocked me down and out for a while, making me almost lethargic. It also knocked me out of any kind of symptoms of euphoric bipolar!

Now as my nerves started pulling back together, I didn't understand why I was there. I had lost touch with reality and did not know what had happened. I got upset and started showing frustration toward a male nurse! My concern is that I needed to get back for a choir rehearsal which I was supposed to be directing! I wanted to leave, and did not seem to understand why I couldn't. In defense of the nurse's perspective, he did not know what I was capable of if I lost my temper and he wasn't going to take a chance on that variable. He called for help to strap me on a gurney and give me a shot! During this process, the nurse put his hand on my Adam's apple; my throat. He wouldn't let go, as if he were threatened by me and he was keeping a 'lid' on my threat.

The tragedy is that the voice, which a few months earlier had sung the toughest and most dramatic tenor solos in Handel's *Messiah* would never be the same again! Because of that unknown nurse holding on to my throat, I would never sing in my high tenor voice again! I would sing again, but never sing high again.

When I got out of the hospital, my life, as I knew it, was back to square one. I had to drop out of school. I had to leave my job and let my dream perish along with the relationships of my new found friends. I had to leave town, regroup, and start my life all over again.

Over the next year, I got started seeing a doctor in central California who had a nutritional approach to medicine. He wanted to solve problems nutritionally before using any kind of pharmaceuticals. I learned a lot from him. Through this doctor I was put on State Disability for one year.

I decided if I am going to receive support for a year, and not allowed to work, I'll go back to school. This is the 'second round' of graduate school. A state university is much less expensive than USC. It was affordable without getting a loan to pay for school. We now reset the eighteen-month 'hour' glass. I had studied about this university in advance. There was a Yale theorist on the faculty to teach musical analysis. I was given a faculty advisor that was a world renowned horn player with a PhD in Music Composition. He had been an editor of a national brass magazine for players of brass instruments. I was signing in to the concentration of Musicology as part of an MA degree in Music. It would take two years to complete the program. State Disability was paying for one year. The first major obstacle was facing the graduate record exam. I don't get along with objective tests that are a mile long. Multiple choice tests only declare what you don't know, not what you do know. This really was a mile long! Sure enough, I did not score very high on the test; definitely not high enough for entrance into this graduate school. I spent time with my graduate advisor talking about it. When he realized I was taking medication to enable me to go to school, he had an idea that I could take a different exam that would be acceptable to the university should I pass it. Sure enough, the professor found an exam that had been created in the state of Ohio. On top of that, he was actually going to give me what we call 'accommodations' in Special Education. This is the first time someone deliberately did it even though at my alma mater, I was given comprehensive, all essay, exams, with which I was highly successful. The accommodations I was given were, to administer the test and give me all the time I needed to finish the test. Guess what? I passed it! Another obstacle hurdled.

My first year seemed to go okay, except for studying musicology. It seemed as though my primary musicology professor expected me to already be a musicologist, rather than molding me into one. When I couldn't get a higher grade than a 'C' with the resident musicologist, it's like 'flunking' out of graduate school.

Not only did I have to try to please the musicologist, I heard he was terminally ill. How much did that fact influence his judgment or his motivation to mentor and teach me? I don't know.

My second year at State University Graduate School carried with it some new stressors, testing my nervous system. My state disability money that supported me the first year 'ran out' after one year; so I had to get a job to support myself in grad school.

In downtown LA, I had signed up with a detective agency to do security work when I was younger. I decided to look for a security company that might give me a job. I found Burns International and they gave me a job working nights at a local newspaper as a security guard. By working nights, it didn't matter what my schedule was at school, it would work. Of course, I would have to get some sleep, somehow, some way. My eighteen-month 'hour glass' was running out in my nervous system, I had to work; I also had seemingly failed to please my most important professor of music history.

My heart was that of a composer, a musicology degree would prepare me to teach music history as well. The private school I had attended when I was younger was losing the music history professor to retirement. I was hoping to replace her.

The part of me that was a composer came to the fore. My faculty adviser was a music composition professor, and I talked him into letting me into an advanced music composition class. I needed to prove myself as a composer. I needed more success. I had analyzed and charted linear structure of Claude Debussy's string quartet. I did get the grade of "B" for it. So I had had some success.

As I jumped into the composition class, it was exciting to me because part of the requirement was that I write projects to be performed at a composition recital. Of course, some of the greatest music compositions ever written may have been sacred in nature, based on the musical parts of the Mass in the Catholic Church,

JS Bach, Mozart, and Beethoven. How public universities cannot acknowledge the sacred genres of music from famous composers, I don't understand. This state university and composition professor had absolutely no problem with my desire to write a setting of Psalm 96 for Soprano and Organ. The professor also had organized an advanced instrumental Group: a Woodwind Quintet. He encouraged me to also write a Woodwind Quintet; which I did. In my development as a composer, both of these compositions were quite important in their own ways. They were successful and both were performed at the composition recital. The Quintet was quite complex in its structure and I needed to ask my professor to conduct it for me at the recital. It was exciting and had organic energy of its own. I was so happy to be able to hear it! It brought me great joy! An organist and an accomplished soprano from my church were only happy to perform my composition based on Psalm 96 by King David of Israel. It was special to have my parents witnessing the performance and hearing the composition recital at state university.

The Quintet included a very successful twelve-tone Canon, a complex juxtaposition of difficult to write techniques from the eighteenth century and the early twentieth century. The Woodwind Quintet of which I speak became the most advanced instrumental piece I had ever written. This was a really important opportunity to prepare to write my first Wind Symphony. I had been inspired by a collection of writings by some renowned 'Ivy League' and Netherland theorists and decided to try some of the ideas including formulating my own way of using twelve-tone counterpoint. If you are a music major, this will mean something to you. Otherwise, don't worry; it is virtually a complicated musical puzzle. It required advanced university or professional musicians to perform it. It would have been tough to play for anyone else. Also, it was very important to my development as a composer.

As I swung into the third semester of graduate school at State U., a cloud of depression was hanging over me. The eighteenth-month 'hour glass' had almost run out of sand.

I had pulled down some grades of 'B' in music theory, Analysis, and composition but no 'A's' and no kind of High grades in music history like I had received as a college Senior.

It had taken almost two years to determine that my objective of getting a degree in musicology or music history was not happening. The depression of having failed myself was setting in, even though I was getting an 'A' going into the final in Eighteenth Century Counterpoint: Canon and Fugue Writing, I blew it by not taking the final exam. I was depressed and ready to leave town! I was too upset to do my final and get my first and only 'A.' My graduate adviser told me he hated to ask me to stay two more years get my grades up and complete a degree in Music Composition. It made an option and he believed I could do it! I walked away to start all over.

At this time, I checked in at my parents again. My younger brother had just graduated from college. We built our dad a nice fence in the backyard of the old home place. That was fun and interesting to build something with him right after he became a construction engineer. I am sure, after that, I got busy driving tractor or harvesting alfalfa on a nearby farm or both for the summer.

I left and moved to the Central Coast. I signed up to be a substitute teacher, mostly public junior high school. Junior High substitute teaching is as tough as any there is. In this particular Central California Coastal town, there was an element of Mexican-American students (especially boys), as hard as any I had seen before or since, even in South Central LA. Their jaws were hard set, 'stone faced.' I wasn't sure how I was supposed to deal with them. I was too naïve to know if they were in a gang. I gave them respect and expected them to give me respect in return, but I didn't know if they would. Later, I found out the principal liked having me there because of those 'hard' kids. I don't know why, because I was playing it by ear.

Another side of this story was from the musician side of me. I heard a junior high band concert with a band director that was retiring. It was rather pitiful. It put a desire in me to make an opportunity for myself to at least have a 'shot' at the job.

I joined a trumpet trio and the Community Concert Band as a soloist. Not only that I was asked to play solo trumpet parts with a

Children's Honor Choir chosen from around the School District. I toured with them around the district to perform and got paid substitute teacher pay. We even performed for the District School Board.

The trumpet trio I had just joined, also played some difficult to perform Mexican Folk music written by Rafael Mendez. I did one more thing to try to 'set myself up' for the junior high band director job. When playing in the Community Band, I got acquainted with local music teachers that were also playing in it. By these connections, I was able to organize a City Youth Band for the summer. We performed at the county fair.

A friend of mine fixed dinner and invited somebody for me to meet. I had no idea! As I got acquainted with this person, I found out, was an Assistant County Superintendent of Schools. He was in charge of Special Education for the whole county. He spent time trying to convince me that I would be good at it, and that there was a future in Special Education for teachers.

Now I had quite a few units of graduate school, but absolutely no state credentials to teach. He was showing me that if I just got started in a credential program, he could help me get a job. Now I had no guarantee of getting the band Director job, because I had graduate school in music but no Credential. I had just tried to make myself known around the Community and a do a good job as a substitute teacher. Believe me I had no idea what the world of special education was all about! I could not relate to the value of the offer to teach Special Education, I did not have a point of reference. I was not ready, as wonderful as it was for my friend to introduce me to the Assistant County Superintendent.

This next summer, I found myself at my parents again working on a farm and applying to a variety of jobs. My heart was into the inner city of South Central LA where I had been before. I was considered and accepted as a youth and music director in a multicultural inner city church.

My endeavor was supported by teaching fourth to fifth grades through the week, on the church grounds. My music director position took off and my work with teenagers took a different direction, even though it was experience nonetheless.

I got elected Vice President of the youth organization for the region from Manhattan Beach all the way to Long Beach and Huntington Beach and up to Norwalk and Downey and all the inner city between them. My goal was to raise the level of the quality of teen activities so that the large church youth groups wanted to participate and the small church youth groups would receive the greatest benefit from that effort. I served in this capacity for two years and felt like I accomplished what I set out to do.

Somewhere in the middle of those years, I left the inner city to again enroll in graduate school at Long Beach State University for a Master's in Musicology.

It was back to graduate school. I spent time analyzing linear construction of a short ballet written by Claude Debussy. This kind of work eventually took me to a PhD Dissertation written about the linear construction in the works of Debussy up to 1910 in relation to his expression as a Symbolist. This was written by a PhD candidate at the University of Southern California.

The premise was that Debussy was more closely related to the Symbolist poets than the Impressionist painters. This musicologist's dissertation inspired me to continue the work this musicologist started. To continue it meant doing a theoretical and historical study of Debussy's works from 1908 to the end of his life. That would be exciting to me, mainly because it would mostly be theoretical (meaning musical analysis).

I started getting acquainted with the music involved. My faculty advisor suggested that I research the composer's spirituality. The composer's personal life wasn't very well known. Was he transcendentalist or what? I began going deep into research and spending many hours in the university library. A friend shared with me a new book on the market at the time, *Holy Blood, Holy Grail*. This was an interesting book, but could not necessarily be trusted as being historically accurate. However, it could be valuable as far as my sensitivity to documented relationships that Debussy was known to have. Debussy was associated with the French Symbolist poets who in turn were part of the occult revival of the mid nineteenth century. Edgar Allen Poe also had an association with them and the occult revival.

What was interesting about all this is that in *Holy Blood, Holy Grail*, Debussy was listed as Grand Master of a secret society of devil worshipers in Paris. Now remember, this is not a proven historical fact, but wasn't in conflict with what we do know about him; an example being an unfinished operatic composition on *The Devil in the Belfry* by Edgar Allen Poe.

The library did have, in English, a copy of what was considered to be the 'bible' of the Occult revival. I read it and remembered some impressions I had of it. It seemed that the trek, through the book, included always a quest for wealth in the form of jewels down in an earthen cavern. It also kept you turned all around that they seek hell, the way Christians seek heaven. Heaven is hell and hell is heaven!

The secret society that Debussy may or may not have been part of, were prominent people down through over one thousand years of history. They also believed they were descendents of Jesus and Mary Magdalene. This secret society supposedly has been amassing wealth for all these hundreds of years.

Why? I have my ideas but they are rather far-fetched from analyzing the complicated music of one of the true innovative Fathers of twentieth century music.

Within the world of Christianity, there could be no greater deception than for wealthy, influential world rulers to believe themselves to be earthly descendents of Jesus. If the claims of Christianity are true that Jesus was really the Son of God, died, was raised from the dead and returned to Heaven to sit at the right hand of the throne of God, as opposed to establishing an earthly family of offspring which goes completely against the claims of the Bible.

This is my question. What if this wealth is being amassed for the end times when an Antichrist is suppose to arise, take over the world and take on supernatural powers from Satan directly? Only God would know that. It would take Satanists to believe one of the biggest lies coming from the father of lies, to believe they were flesh and blood descendents of Jesus. They would have had to believe he did not die, and was not raised from the dead. He was not the Son of God, at least in the way Christians believe him to be part of the plan of salvation for humanity.

A couple years later, I had moved away making it harder to get to school, especially on a rainy day. I was supposed to analyze a score of music by another early twentieth century innovator, Arnold Shoenberg. I could not even find a copy of the score in the UCLA Music Library, and couldn't get a hold of my professor to tell him.

At the time, I had married a woman with three kids and was working as a substitute teacher for the county system of court schools. One day, when I really had to make it to graduate school and tell my professor about not being able to find my score to analyze, we had a rain storm. It was impossible to trek across the entire LA basin in a rain storm in a given amount of time after working all day at camp!

I had to examine my own heart. My heart was that of a composer. I did enjoy historical research and analyzing music. Musicology as a field was only going to prepare to teach college level music history and theory. My other consideration was this, I don't need to continue the work of a musicologist that he started in his PhD dissertation and walk away myself, with only a Master's degree and a Master's Thesis in musicology. Way too much work!

It was my choice to quit musicology this time. I needed to get back to my academic 'first love,' Music Composition. During my time at Long Beach State U, I had started my first symphony for Concert Band and also started converting Psalm 96 into a concert choir composition. The University Choir hummed through it for me. The professor/conductor was also an editor for a choral pub- lisher. I was, of course, hoping he would be interested in helping me get it published. When I decided to quit musicology, I found a state university closer to home in which I enrolled to study graduate level music composition.

The Advanced Music Composition Professor liked the idea of me writing a new Movement II for my Band Symphony as my class project. I did it. More than one of my composition professors consid- ered it my best writing yet! I also took a film composition class under the Head of CBS Television Music Dept. That was fun! We had to write four sections of movie score on which our professor had written the original score. We had access to the University Studio Orchestra. We could write for any instrument or any group of instruments, and we did. That was cool! The next semester, I finished the last move-ment to my symphony and wrote a mini-opera for male quartet, brass quartet, and string quartet named, *Moses and Pharaoh.*

My creative juices were really flowing at a high level. I was hav-ing success, straight A's in graduate level Music Composition. If I stayed with it, the degree I could receive would be Master of Music in Composition. All this was very stimulating academically! Hang on! I had to walk away. My eighteen-month 'hour' glass seemed to be running out; but that isn't why I walked away.

I had to consider a different direction as far as making a living, since I had three 'ready-made' children and a 'home- made' daughter by then. Supporting a family was going to have to take precedence over my development as a composer.

When we got married, I was working on a boys' ranch. The boys were placed there by the juvenile court judges. These boys had lives that were messed up, but at a stage where they didn't have to be locked up any more or yet, they just had to serve time in an 'open placement' to please the judge. I finally got skilled enough at work-ing with these teens that I was in charge of them if they got 'kicked out' of school for behavior issues. So, I had to be there during school hours, not to mention making sure they were up and ready for school with the ranch house cleaned inside and out before school. I had worked with youth in churches and youth organizations for activi-ties, music, drama, athletic endeavors, and even a little teaching in private or Christian schools; but never 'troubled' teens. This is where I transition towards being an educator of difficult to manage. There was considerable graduate school involved in teacher education in California to establish a career in it, also enabling me to help raise and support five children.

PART II

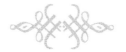

Career Building

8

To Build a Career

I learned a lot at the boys' ranch, and got the idea to start working as a substitute teacher. Gradually, by experience, I learned the importance of constant supervision to these kinds of teens. At the extreme north end of Los Angeles County, on the edge of the Mojave Desert, is where the boys' ranch was located. The county sent two teachers out there to establish two classrooms. At some point, I got acquainted with the assistant principal who passed through periodically and I found out about substitute teaching for the county. Meanwhile, I had another job besides week day wake-up and school-time counseling and discipline of students that got sent out of class. Every Friday, I loaded up a large van with boys that, by good behavior, had earned a home visit. I took them to the very heart of South Central LA, the inner city. Every week at the end of the weekend, on Sunday night, I would go get the boys and bring them back up to the ranch where we would have to search them carefully to make sure they didn't bring some drugs.

A couple of these trips were memorable for the drama they held. One of the boys was in a gang and went to visit his girlfriend that was in rival gang territory and was stuck. He had to figure out how to get out of there without getting shot by the enemy! So, he wasn't

45

back from his ordeal when I went to pick him up. He finally got out of there alive, but I couldn't wait for him that night!

I remember talking to a fifteen year old, small of stature, "Mr. Cool." He was soft spoken and very confident. We were standing in the hallway of the large ranch house that housed twenty-five boys. He told me about his dreams for the future. He wanted to live in a big house, as a gangster, untouchable by the cops. Wow! What a dream! I had worked for an inner city church for a time in gang territory and as an officer in a youth organization where I had developed a great deal of compassion for those involved in gangs. This time, a fifteen-year-old was standing in front of me, calm, quiet, and respectful. I really liked him. Not very long after that, I took him for a home visit down to the middle of LA. I didn't think much about it at the time, because I did it every week. Sunday night, I went to pick him up and he was not there! He did not even reach his sixteenth birthday! He took a gang-related bullet and did not survive! The reality of gang life hit closer to my heart than I had ever experienced before!

At the other end of the spectrum, I remember a rather amazing story told by the president and owner of West Coast Detectives two or three years earlier. The occasion, I was there to get a job. When I was in college, a number of years earlier and was strong from weight lifting for the track team, I had worked security detail for West Coast Detectives. When I had to go back to school, the owner of West Coast Detectives told me to come back if I ever needed a job. Well, I did. They ushered me into the office of the Head of West Coast Detectives. The ownership had changed hands and this owner was a dynamic Christian! I told him I had been working with inner city youth, and had a great deal of concern for them and those involved in gangs; but I needed a job.

He said that he would give me a job; then he proceeded to tell me a story. Members of a street gang had gathered in a park located within their 'turf,' a place where they 'hung out' fairly often. This time was different. A visitor was with them and had been sharing from the bible to them and was starting to pray with them for their spiritual renewal and salvation. Suddenly, one of their fiercest rival gangs completely surrounded them! Just as suddenly, they ran away mysteriously frightened as if they had seen ghosts! Later, when some-one asked the question of the intruders to what had happened here was the explanation: as the other gang was bowing to pray, they were completely surrounded by angels! Any other gang would have been scared and turn to run away! That's what happened, right here in South Central LA.

That was one story I could never forget! So I had to share it here! While I still worked at the boys ranch and had remarried, I woke up to a brand new adventure one morning! I was awake because I had to get up to go to work. Then I heard the words floating from the restroom: 'My water broke.' My wife was famous, in the family, for delivering babies really fast; but this was my very first one! I just knew I better get her to the hospital as soon as possible! I remember seeing the doctor on the way, in his big Classic Cadillac convertible. When we got to the street the hospital was on, leave it to me to not turn and keep on going. I had to find a place to hang a U-turn and get back on my way to the hospital! That did add a comical element to the story, that no one will let me forget, by the way! Sure enough, my wife's water broke at 6:20am and delivered a nine-pound baby at 7:20am. I am sure my first baby would be a boy because of her size alone. The nurse put her in my arms and said I had myself a musician instead of a football player! When I took her into arms for the very first time, I was perfectly happy with that!

Sometime during that rushed morning I had to let my super-visor know I wouldn't be at work as usual. Later in the morning I called him from the hospital room while holding my baby daughter and looking over the city from the third floor up. He was begging me to come to work. I was so proud of that baby; I did not want to stop holding her for anything; even to go to work

As I got the opportunity to start substitute teaching for LA County Juvenile Court Schools, the benefits included that they were year round schools. They also offered higher pay than any small local districts. It was important to learn from permanent teachers, the pro-cedures and 'tricks' to help keep classrooms under control and avoid the kinds of problems these 'hardcore' students could cause for a substitute teacher.

One of the first things to do was following the lesson plans the teacher left and grading the work as needed. It was important to follow seating charts, make sure all pencils were accounted for and move around the room to make sure students were not 'tagging' or doing gang-related writing.

Allowing students to engage in any gang-related communication can lead to a fight rather quickly. It was imperative to stay on top of the development of any kind of disruption or provocation between students in the classroom. Keeping students absolutely 'on quiet' was very helpful.

The toughest place to do all this seemed to be at Juvenile Hall. If I could do all these things and produce a good amount of work through the students, it was possible to impress the permanent teacher. If the regular teacher liked your work, you were occasionally asked to cover the teacher again or even a vacation.

These teachers were on a twelve-month contract and so they could ask for vacation days most anytime throughout the year. It was attractive to me that these teachers went to work and left as soon as school was out, seemingly done with their day, and ready to walk away. Some teachers had a system of keeping up with their paperwork throughout the day including daily grades.

I am sure there was planning on the part of the teachers that I didn't see. I am sure that some had a systematic way of teaching a discipline that made easy to go in, do it and leave. This looked good to me not knowing that I would ever get a permanent job in a camp for myself. I had a lot to experience before that could happen.

As I was supporting four children, I got called to work almost everyday. I got paid by the day, but had no benefits for my family. I would go most anywhere in North County to work. I got the idea to sign up for substitute teaching in the Division of Special Education for the County as well.

It would ensure that I would have a place to work everyday. My problem was that I did not know anything about Special Ed. At the time, the County Special Education sites were on the campuses of regular education schools but dealt with mostly severe handicaps of which there was a variety. There were developmentally delayed or retardation to deal with. Deaf and hard of hearing usually had their own classrooms. Autistic students, Including a variety of physical handicaps, were part of a list of different kinds of that we needed to be able to step in and work with. There was a severe handicap that was closer to the kind of students with which I was used to working. It was the severely emotionally disturbed

There were always teacher assistants in these classrooms, which we now call paraeducators. As I started, I had no idea what I was doing. I was following the leadership of the paraeducators and learning all I could from these patient and wonderful people. At the time, they were God-sent to me. I knew so little about special education, the paraeducator or the assistant principal would mention that I was good with a certain kind of student and I didn't understand what was meant because I didn't know anything about these students or their educational needs. At the time I didn't know what 'good' referred to. This was a whole new world to me. My dad would call it a 'whole new ballgame.'

My experiences in special education and my knowledge of the workings of special education grew slowly as I got calls to 'sub' in those classrooms intermingled with incarcerated youth of the County Probation Camp Schools.

Part of my education included a degree in Fine Arts-Music. The Fine Arts 'part' entailed drama and histories of various forms of art and architecture. I remember one of the first times I wanted to let the students do a little art and use colored pencils. I had to count the pencils and make sure they all got back before the incarcerated student left the classroom. I also pulled the blue and red pencils, or made sure anyone using blue had to use red as well. Red and Blue would be targeted for being stolen. Blue would be targeted for being stolen. I had to handle it strictly and carefully to avoid problems. I was with boys back in those days there were a lot of gang related issues with enemies like Bloods and Crips. I had to be circulating around the room with eyes peeled to observe someone doing gang-related writing or art work. In this situation, I wanted some moments of creativity for my students but I was learning that I had to do it carefully and deliberately.

Gang-related rivalry had no place in my classroom, that is, if I wanted to survive! This was on-the-job training; everyday was 'survival of the fittest.' I had to be the fittest because I had a family at home to support. Any time I could discover enemy 'gang bangers' within my classroom it was to my advantage, so that I could find a way to avoid conflicts. If they peacefully co-existed in my classroom without my knowledge that was great! It meant they were busy being students.

The challenge to be a substitute teacher was to have a way of convincing students that you wouldn't tolerate gang-related 'anything' in the classroom. One lever to be articulated would be that a judge would add 'time' to their stay. It just so happens a quick communication to 'put down' another's hood can explode to violence at the 'drop-of-a-hat'!

Suddenly, I was being ushered in into lives of inner city kids, some of whom were hardcore of 'gangbangers.' This had been a prayer of mine, a desire, but God had his own way of preparing me for it and playing it out in my life. This was the beginning.

It was helpful to my development to be able to take over a class while a teacher was on vacation. There was a small placement up a canyon road, somewhat like a boys ranch that required three County teachers. It was not a 'locked' facility like a camp. If students did not do well there, the judge might send them to a probation camp.

During the time I was covering a vacation, I came up with some creative writing projects that opened the hearts and imaginations of these young men. It was touching to see the amazing talent just for free-verse poetry!

Then I concocted a plan to have a 'rap' contest. Raps can be ballads of street life including drugs, gangs, sex, and violence. I had to create rules that students would 'buy' into and still be motivated to rap. Here was the plan, students had to create a rap for young children, brother, sister, cousin. The rap had to be positive; an encouragement for kids to avoid the life of being in a gang or harmful consuming of drugs in the streets. This rap would be a warning to children and would be free of profanity or any kind of sex talk altogether. Guess what? It worked! They went for it in a noble competition! Some, I would have been proud to have broadcast on the radio for kids to hear!

Another time, I got asked to be a substitute teacher at a probation camp. It would be for two weeks of a teacher's vacation. I taught Biology and one other core subject like Civics. I was with each class for two subjects. Then I switched two more times adding up to six periods of high school.

I am only mentioning it at this time, because of the academic game I created. Of course, this book is meant to be an encouragement to teachers. You are welcome to utilize any innovations you find herein. I used them on Friday to review what the students were supposed to have learned through the week.

1) The teacher has to prepare questions based on the week's chapter (ahead of time) on 3x5 cards, folded once with question inside.

2) Teacher picks two captains that are responsible and good academically. Captains choose up teams and pick the name of their team. If it is related to sports teams, that adds a shot of enthusiasm and motivation, depends on sports season football or basketball, it helps to use it for scoring points. For my model of explanation we will choose football.

3) Each team will sit in a circle so they can discuss the question and decide as a team what the best answer is.
   This takes the pressure off individual students that don't know answers, but it will help them learn. If a person blurts out the wrong answer the turn goes to the other team (just like some sports change ball possession). You can't score unless you have the ball. In this case, the 'ball' is the question.)

4) Like a real game, flip a coin to see which team goes first. Hold a handful of folded 3x5 cards, folds up. Ask the captain to choose a question by pulling one out randomly. (Do not open). Hand question to teacher. Both teams in

huddles consider the answer; as question is read orally by the teacher

5) A detail you can add: if the answer has two parts and the First team gets one part they score ½ a touchdown or three points like a 'field goal.' If the other team comes up with the remainder of the answer also score three points

The first two Fridays I used this game while the teacher was on vacation the competition became so intense! You could imagine a real football game between them; except they were using brains only!

If you are a teacher reading this, feel free to use this game to livin' up a Friday or as a chapter review for older students. This is non-intimidating for the students who didn't study, it's a good way to draw them in.

As I expanded my horizons of education to include special education students that needed a substitute teacher, I began to find out the kinds of students for which I was better suited. To remind you of the practical side of this, if the Court Schools didn't need a 'sub,' I would have a better chance of working everyday if I was signed up for north county special education classrooms.

I remember a particular situation out of town where I got an opportunity to work with a ten or eleven-year-old boy that was severely emotionally disturbed. I was given a room in which to work with him. He came from a classroom full of emotionally disturbed taught by a County special education teacher. He was the worst behaved student on a mission to drive his teacher crazy, or so it seemed. He had a serious problem with impulse control. In that larger class, he was out of control. He was disrespectful. He was defiant of almost anything the teacher asked him to do. He would walk across the top of desks. All the other students were at their desks doing what they were suppose to do. So, the rest of the students may have been classified emotionally disturbed but they seemed to have, for the most part, bought in to the program.

For me, this became a long term Sub Teacher position. That was great! For my family, it was a little stability knowing where I was going to work everyday, even if it was only for awhile. During my observation of this boy, I noticed that the teacher's and/or the paraeducator's approach to him 'set-him-off.' He had a very 'short fuse' and negative attention was just as important to him as if he were getting praise for bad behavior. By taking our student out of there, it took away the audience for which he was performing (his mates); and I was going to deal with him in such a way as to not 'set-him-off'.

My plan was to be consistently strict, quiet-mannered, and not show emotion if I had to discipline the student. Be clear about rules and then set up a positive reinforcement system into which he could buy.

Since he was in the mode of running-his-own-program, the positive reinforcements had to be set for one assignment at a time or short intervals of a half-hour. My success with him was fairly dramatic! The administration started sending me other students that weren't 'making it' where they were. We had our own room out of which to operate and the start of the next semester of school they would bring in a permanent, veteran teacher to take over the class we were establishing.

It was helpful to have the student one-on-one for a little while and establish a wide range of dimensions to our relationship. To give you an idea, I had coached several sports in the past; so I tuned into his athleticism using P.E. time to better his skills. Boys at this age, are very sensitive to their abilities or lack there of, and want to learn various athletic skills to save ridicule by others, ridicule by others, as well as being motivated to hone skills in their favorite sport.

Another area in which I was able to use, to help mellow out my relationship with this student and motivate him to want to be in school, was through music. I was able to teach him simple fundamentals of music and to read music with a student recorder. Some band directors use this as a pre-band instrumental music activity. Because of my degree in music and my music teaching experience, I was able to have creative ways of using music as incentives for finishing assignments or earning time to listen to music among others. As you hear of 'music to calm the beast,' I learned in the early days of my work with students having emotional disturbance it was even more important in a therapeutic sense.

Somehow I had established a bit of a reputation for myself in the North County with special education students. One of the first principals I had met in the court schools when I first started 'subbing' for the county crossed my path and told me he had become a special education principal.

His comment was that he had heard of my good work and that he wanted to get me working back up near home in his special education area. This was great to know, administrators were taking notice and starting to believe in my abilities with special needs children. Teachers started to ask me to cover their vacations and work me in long-term 'sub' jobs more and more. My eighteen-month 'hour glass' must have been getting way over due for my bi-polar episode. The chronology of this episode may not be quite accurately lined up with the success I was having in my substitute teaching. I just know that getting straight 'A's' in graduate level advanced music composition added fuel for my next bipolar episode. When the manifestation of my episodes took the euphoric route, intellectual stimulation plays into it more often than not. Also, before I left Long Beach State, I got as far as a Master's Thesis Proposal that was accepted before I had to leave. This also lends some fuel for my episode. You will understand more soon.

Previously, a number of my bipolar episodes were subsequent to something positive or an exciting happening in my life that was stimulating to my mind or heart or both. This set a stage not for major depression, but on the contrary, the euphoric swing of my bipolar.

I was continually looking for supplement work to add to my substitute teaching to increase my bring-home pay. I spent a little while making hamburgers at McDonald's and selling men's clothing at a clothing store. This particular time, I was looking for a part-time sales position that would help me better support my family.

9

Last Major Nervous Breakdown!

I had found one. My hour glass had run out! I was starting to have my last major nervous breakdown! Considering my condition had never been properly diagnosed! Then any medications I took were only a temporary fix. Their effectiveness ran out.

A few years earlier, Prudential had recruited me to sell insurance and other adjacent products. They required a college graduate. I was one. They were ready to back me launching a career. It came down to this; I had to pass the state generated tests that would license me to sell insurance.

Back to back objective tests, multiple choice questions a half a mile long and only so much time to do it. Well, I missed the required score to pass by a few questions on both tests. I would rather have a three-hour comprehensive essay in musicology any day.

Why am I bringing this up now? For some reason these people did believe in my ability to become a salesman. So I guess it kind of went to my head. It started me believing I could do it.

I pursued another sales job, and was accepted. They were getting me to believe I could make $10,000 per month. All I had to do was get supermarkets or any store with shopping carts where there could be placed ads and a small directory to show locations of certain goods in the store.

One of my first assignments took me out of town about ninety miles up the edge of the desert. I was already losing touch with reality. I was going to get 'rich' fast. I believed that so much, I had tires put on my wife's car, for which it was way overdue. I bought a light high-powered rifle to give my stepson for big game hunting. I had worked with him and supported him in completing a hunter safety course needed to get a hunting license. To show how out of touch with reality I was by using money in the bank that was for rent. I guess it was not unusual for bipolar to show euphoric symptoms by needless and illogical spending.

Another thing I did that was really out of touch was to write a letter to a former music professor that had become academic dean at the small Christian college I had attended when I was young. A Dean is the one that hires professors. My letter said I was working on a PhD with a double concentration, Music Composition and Musicology at a specific campus of the University of California. After all, I finished my Symphony For Band and a Mini Opera. I could write an opera for the Dissertation. My alma mater's musicologist said he would help me get into that school if I really wanted to go and finish the Master's Thesis proposal Debussy's music for doctoral Dissertation in Musicology. It was honestly too much work for a Master's degree. That was the thinking behind writing my former professor. I knew he was going to need someone to teach Music History.

Of course, the university where I could get these PhD's was located on the Central Coast and the school where I always wanted to teach was located on the South Coast, and I had not even applied to the PhD school, let alone starting to even work on such a degree except to USC a number of years earlier. All of these were perhaps possible someday, but I wasn't a music professor ready to report right now. I started doing strange things in the front yard. My wife called a mental health service that would come out and evaluate me free of charge in case I needed to go to the county hospital. When it was mentioned that I bought a gun, the local sheriff immediately got me in the hospital eventually moving me to a county hospital. Seventy-two hrs is mandatory, but two weeks if I agree and sign myself in to stay.

My oldest (step)children, bless their hearts, drove all the way back up there to take the rifle back to the gun shop, and made a deal with the tire man to pay off the tires, so they could get some of that money back. To this day, it is embarrassing to hear what they had to do. Every time I got this ill in my past, my life blew apart! In fact, any significant other I had in my life at that time... vanished! Anything good I had going for myself fell apart, and I had to start my life all over somewhere else!

This was different. My wife said I asked her why she was there (while at the hospital for a visit). I remember peering out the window from high in the hospital and seeing all the children down by the car, even though they probably didn't get to visit.

This hospital is where they finally diagnosed me correctly as bipolar disorder. They were realizing they had to find the right medication for me. After all these many years with medicine that was only a temporary 'fix,' maybe they could find something more effective.

The Doctors told my wife that my illness was so serious that she could walk away from me! They also told her that my IQ put me at some level of genius. Praise the Lord, I had someone that did not give up on me for the first time in my life! (besides my mother of course)

10

Regrouping

I could not go back to work for a while and spent time trying medicine until I got the best therapeutic level using the most effective 'stuff.' I started out with Lithium, which I had tried once before. Lithium had become a good, effective medicine for bipolar. It was actually a salt-like substance already in the body and the doctor just increases the level. For me it made me too slow and sluggish. Eventually, Tegretol worked better. It's hard to believe I went through all this since seventeen to finally have a medicine that helped me manage life and stressful jobs. I had a wife and a whole family that never gave up! That's amazing!

It only took a doctor's release to go back to work and go back to my development as an educator. As if to seal the confidence of my little family that wouldn't give up on me, a new addition was on the way, and I was back to work building the confidence of school administrators as well.

My youngest daughter had an appointment to be delivered on the last Saturday in September. We were suppose to meet at the hospital at 8am and prepare to spend all day as the birth would be induced. I held my wife's hand all day. The college football season had started, my favorite season of the year. Since my wife wouldn't have felt much like watching TV in her hospital room, I watched some football on her behalf as I held her hand.

Within a year of her being born, I was offered a job in special education working for the county. This was exciting because my family would be finally covered by benefits!

It was unusual, in that, you had to have at least a preliminary credential to be a teacher in charge of a classroom in California. I had a graduate school, but absolutely no credential schooling. An attorney came from county headquarters to go through the formality of presenting me a waver (of credential) for me to take over a classroom immediately. Since they went to so much trouble to put me to work with severely emotionally disturbed; then I had to sign-up in a hurry for a teacher training program. As I did I decided, I needed to work on a multiple subject credential and start taking special education classes toward a special education credential as well. The multiple subject prepared one to teach all core subjects in the state curriculum.

This was amazing! My administrator believed in me and went to a lot of trouble to give me a job. A former college of mine took me immediately into their Teacher Education Program! My wife and family didn't give up on me and I had a beautiful one year old daughter of my very own.

One of the toughest teaching jobs there is, happens to be junior high-aged with severe emotional disturbance. This age is squirrellier than high school-aged and the impulsive behaviors are more extreme. An example would be leaving out of the room and climbing up on the roof.

The precarious situation, in which we find ourselves, is like this; location of the classroom was adjacent to the junior high school overseen by the County Superintendent of Schools. The students, the staff on the regular education campus, and possibly the surrounding community may observe extreme impulsive behaviors. The first response you would expect them to have is, why don't you have your students under control? Considering we just got the student, so we barely know him at all; it will take time to modify extreme behavior. The people that could be 'up-in-arms,' would not know nor understand this.

Another dimension of this has to do with an important reason to be adjacent to a regular education school. A goal of special education is to equip and enable students to 'mainstream' back into regular education even if it is little by little, ideally insuring success to the student. It was important to find the strength that a student has and give moral support to the point of risking her or him in a regular education school knowing it could back-fire! On the other hand, it may be worth the risk if he or she is successful.

By the time our students get to us, their failures immensely out weigh any successes. Their self-esteem and confidence in themselves are registered at 'E,' like a gas tank out of gas. I am sure we will talk about these a great deal later in these writings. We have come across athletes with above average skill. In some of graduate research later on, I discovered the findings of psychologists on the East Coast claiming there are three times as many gifted or talented students found among troubled or incarcerated youth as compared to regular education population.

During my substitute teaching years, I was fortunate to be able to spend time with and 'sub' for the best teachers in the county. I easily took the 'tricks' of the trade wherever I went and they worked for me.

One simple strategy required you to get to know your students a little bit. What are some of their interests outside of school? Motorcycles? Sports? Music? Entertainment? As a teacher, I am going to want to get them started reading. Also, I am going to want to make them read quietly at a certain time everyday. So my plan is to round up high-interest magazines to get them started, even the students that don't want to read at all. If you have special day class students, they will be in your room all day for all subjects. Then you want to collect a classroom library as you can, always listening for clues to students interests that could help you get them started reading books.

When we got a more permanent teacher to take the junior high emotionally disturbed class, the assistant principal then wanted me to see what kind of impact my music skills could have on an autistic class. At various times in the past, in fairly recent history, music had miraculous results with autism by impacting communication or uncovering amazing musical talent. My boss knew I was a composer; she wanted to see what I could do.

I did come up with musical responses that were interesting. I was given a 'so-called' junior high aged autism class but there were a variety of handicaps, and only minimum communication through simple sign language. We had a speech pathologist and a psychologist who were critical to planning communication and behavior strategies for the teacher to implement in the classroom. They were really important to me, present were mental retardation developmentally delayed, fetal alcohol syndrome, and cerebral palsy.

One student was twelve years old, but had never been 'potty trained.' During 'music time' I noticed his interest in music. We got out various percussion and rhythm instruments. I either played the piano or put on music album for the students to play along. I had brought over a real snare drum from the junior high school next door. It was especially exciting for the one that needed 'potty' training.

I got the idea to use the drum as an incentive for making progress with this boy's 'potty training.' I timed it so I could start setting up music instruments, at the same time he was set to the restroom on the toilet. I cracked the door to the restroom so he could see what I was doing. My student did not want to miss music time so he had results on the toilet. That was amazing! No one had results like that with him before! It was hard to sustain over a long period of time to get maximum results in the restroom; but it was quite noteworthy to mention here.

Another significant impact that music had on this class was self-abuse. One twelve-year-old Down syndrome boy was in a helmet most of the time because of self-abuse. He would hit his forehead with the back of his fist until his head started bleeding His helmet fit down far enough to cover his forehead. That helped.

I learned that when he started hitting himself, if I would go sit at the piano and start playing he would immediately stop the self-abuse and he would come and sit by me on the piano bench. It was rather amazing what music did for him!

I had one more self-abuser. He was tall, junior high-aged, and would sit on the floor backed up against the wall. He was more autistic as he rocked back and forth resembling autistic stemming. He would bite his wrist as part of that stemming until he bled. His wrists had to be wrapped up in bandages, enough to make it harder for him to bite. I did have a classroom record player when this boy started biting his wrists. I put on a record album of the trumpet player, Doc Severinsen. He immediately stopped biting when he heard the jazz trumpet album. It was the only album that was 'magic.' I experimented with all different kinds of music albums. That one worked immediately every time!

These were the most impressive results to therapy with music that I recall from teaching that autism class. At the end of the school year there were eminent teacher cutbacks across the state with the most students.

For my family, it was a bit of a disaster. After all of the years of being a substitute teacher without benefits, now I finally have benefits and we are facing teacher cutbacks! A teacher from another side of the county with completed credentials wanted my job and my class. Meanwhile, I have only a partial credential, which I felt terribly insecure when teachers are being laid off. We were finally in our own home and have a little apartment on the back for my wife's grandmother, but we lost it all unable to make payments.

Finally, I went into the edge of Los Angeles and got a job teaching students with emotional disturbance in a psychiatric care facility for high school-aged students. I was offered a job teaching the kind of students I wanted to teach. It was a non-public school so it couldn't demand the full credentials. It also couldn't pay the salary. I used the opportunity for experience and to finish my credentials and a master's degree. My salary was lower, but it was steady work for my family's sake with at least some benefits. My university was giving me on-the-job credit and monitoring by my faculty advisor.

I was working on multiple credentials. I was working on a Multiple Subject K-12; Learning Handicapped, along with a Certificate to Teach Severe Emotional Disturbance. So, the focus of my Master's Degree in Education was on severe emotional disturbance, which many times were accompanied by lesser handicaps or processing disorders. Our school had all emotionally disturbed students and it was an open placement where they lived and got full psychological services and social workers to advocate for the students and provide group therapy.

Our school may not have been a public school, but it got its students from Los Angeles Unified; therefore if there was an important meeting or a special education meeting concerning the student, there was always a representative from LA Unified present, usually a psychologist.

The credentials I was working on was perfect for this kind of work. My Multiple Subject was needed as my classes were self-contained and I taught them all day, all subjects. My Learning Handicapped was important; not knowing what student might come in class with more than one type of difficulty in learning. A Severe Emotional Disturbance Certificate allowed me to move over from mild and moderate classifications to a severe area of handicapping condition.

The psychiatric care facility was an entity unto itself. It contracted a corporation to manage the school. It sounds kind of funny, but it was to my advantage. I learned a lot. It was very well run and had administrators with earned doctoral degrees in education.

A great deal of training was provided for the kind of students we were about to teach. I had mentioned before, that these students had been overloaded with negative experiences in their lives. For so long, their self-worth was about 'knee high' to a grasshopper. This company had their own way of helping with that:

1) Avoiding any unnecessary negative redirection.
2) Constantly showering everyone with positive input for good behavior, for good work, for good focusing, for ignoring negative input and not feeding into negative behavior.
3) Finding positive input to give all around the person that is caught up in negative attitudes and behavior. Teacher hopes the student will want positive attention instead of not caring if the attention is negative or positive.

4) A near exaggeration of positives around the classroom constantly may feel 'funny' at first; but it reaps wonderful results in changing culture and atmosphere.

An administrator would observe classrooms very often to make sure the positives were part of the teaching. The administrators in the company had earned doctorates in education. Everything about what we did was governed by educators with high levels of expectations.

This fit into my life and career so well, and learn much that would be valuable later. The graduate advisor for my master's degree met my boss and observed me on the job so as to give me credit for my teaching experiences. To my advantage, I used students' social workers/therapists as if they were my 'parents.' I felt free to go to them and talk to them about my students and give them updates on the students' progress bad or good. I also talked strategies with the therapists that would be helpful in my classroom and in order to keep us on the same page.

My classrooms were all boys. Some of my students were 'gang-bangers' and I had to keep a close eye on those that were in opposing gangs so I could direct them away from conflict. To these students, I enjoyed teaching WWI and WWII. After describing the scenario out of which grew the wars, I picked a corner of the room to decorate and devote to the war. Included were students' research manifested in drawings, and writings about weapons and technical advancements as well as uniforms. I threw in model airplanes and model warships, knowing that if they got built, the risk was high to be destroyed. Students with emotional disturbances, many times, have the shortest fuses for the hottest tempers! I took my chances. The models that the boys did build, I was sure to find documentaries that illustrated their roles in the particular war or part of the war in which they were used (sharing the videos with the rest of the class of course).

Each teacher in this school was expected to take Professional Assault Response Training periodically. The county had its own similar training for Crisis Intervention that included more strategies in 'heading-off' escalations in the classrooms. One, of course, is tuning into your students and their frustrations so much that you can direct them away from losing their temper, especially against somebody.

It became real important to learn to keep tabs on the kind of language that is the most annoying or provocative, and be able to stop it before it turns into something. Moving students to the opposite ends of the classroom sometimes works. Anything to avoid escalation was worth a try. Another idea might be to 'time-out' a student without consequences; this is an opportunity to 'cool-off' and pull themselves together. In a probation camp, I had a probation officer outside the classroom that could talk to them, or in the psychiatric care facility there sometimes was a behavior aide. I made it very clear there would be no consequences at all for the time-outs, especially for the students' sake.

The person that seemed to want to go out of their way to provoke a fight inspired me to go out of my way to make sure it didn't 'come-to-blows' and that the person provoking, got full consequences.

When I was young, slim, and getting ready for college football, I was over two hundred pounds. So I have been big even when I wasn't fat. My metabolism is such that it seems too easy to collect fat if I don't partake in some vigorous exercise. So I'm always pretty big. The last several years of my career I devoted to an all girls' probation camp for the county. I had a student in my class that was bigger than I was, probably three hundred pounds. Somehow she got caught up in provoking another student, they exchanged 'trash talking,' and perpetuated the problem. The big girl was so strong I was about to find out why I later thought she could take on the state high school heavyweight boys wrestling champion! Well, she finally lost it!

There was no holding back now! The scene included a teacher's desk that was near the only entrance to the classroom. The object of the big girl's anger was a slender wisp of a girl, hardly over a hundred pounds. There was no way I could let this best student I ever had, in any school, at any time be attacked! She was a treasure to this teacher's heart! I directed the little one to behind my desk so that there was a 'two-ton' metal teacher's desk between her and the livid 'big' girl. I had to play this just right. When the big girl lunged, but didn't go over my desk, only endangered my computer. I directed the slim girl to quick, get out of the door! I stuck my head out to get help! Probation officers came running. Thankfully, my 'big' girl kept lumbering on out the door before she destroyed my classroom! It took three male probation officers to subdue her. That day, I thought I earned a great deal of respect from the probation officers with my effort to hold off a horrible fight.

If we could return to the psychiatric care facility, I'll tell another dramatic story from my classroom. The facility we were using for this youth center was formerly a county hospital. The classrooms were on the bottom floor with living and recreational areas on the floors two and three. I had a class of all boys. Any girls in the facility were kept separate ninety-eight percent of the time. Because these were teens with emotional handicaps, making a difference would be much harder with hormones and the opposite sex in the equation.

For this teacher tale, we were in a weird-shaped room in a corner. It was a long rectangle with one entrance in the corner and no windows; just inside the door to the right there was a bookcase. Behind the bookcase were the only light switches to the classroom. When the door was closed, it was totally black in the room even though it was the middle of the day. The student desks in the room were the kind that the desk was attached to the seat. My class was of all boys, classified as emotionally disturbed. They were high school-aged, mostly fully-grown. I had a behavior aide assigned to my class-room. He was out of the room at the moment. I was located fairly near the door. One of the closest students to me grabbed a book and threw it against the wall above the bookcase; it perfectly slid down the wall, and turned off the lights making it pitch black! Then he picked up a whole student desk and threw it at me! At the Exact same instant that he picked up the desk, my behavior aide opened the door and streamed in light so he could witness who threw the desk! Because it was pitch black, I did not know a desk was coming at me! It left a bruise below my waste. A city police officer came to arrest him for assaulting a teacher. I did not know how bad my injury was for awhile. Of course they fixed the light to be on and not controlled by a light switch in the room.

When I finally finished my requirements for degree Master's in Education with concentration in Special Education, I also made all my state teaching credentials more permanent. They included a Multiple Subjects K-12 Grades, Learning Handicapped Credential, and a Certificate to Teach Severely Emotionally Disturbed. My multiple subjects credential covered all core subjects up to twelfth grade plus physical education as well. This one, I had difficulty getting. First of all, I had to take a National Teacher's Exam. To pass, I had to get so many correct of a huge objective multiple choice test. I missed two or 3 too many out of six hundred or so, and failed the whole test. My personal feelings about these kind of tests are that they only measure what you don't know, not what you do know; unlike my graduate level musicology exams that were three hours of all essay in which I received a grade of 'A'. If my memory serves me correctly, I took the multiple subjects exam again and failed it again by one or two questions! That was devastating! As a result, I had somebody analyze my transcripts. I was told if I took a couple classes in history and social science, even at the community college level, I would qualify for the credential without even taking the test. I took Sociology and Twentieth Century Europe. Sociology was fairly easy and I loved Twentieth Century Europe! I finally qualified! Twentieth Century Europe class came in handy when I was teaching students about the World Wars. It was a choice for which I was grateful. While I was at the youth center as a teacher, I had a class of all boys. Everything I learned was going to be valuable on my next assignment, and even help me get my next job.

11

The Perfect Job!

Not too often in my life did I ever pray for a particular job. Usually, I asked the Lord to close doors and open the right one. This was different. Now that I had a master's degree in my back pocket, the County Office of Education (COE) would pay me more than anyone (any other school district) if I could find the right job.

COE had a job available at a day treatment center. It was a collaboration between mental health department and office of education. Back when I was a substitute teacher, the most severely handicapped students in every district in the county were taught by county teachers. This little school had only students with severe emotional disturbance. Uniquely, part of the structure included mental health therapists that were on the campus and available throughout the school day as needed. It was a great concept of operation. I loved the setup!

I went back home and started praying to get this job. I was given an interview with several. Before this, I didn't like being interviewed by a committee; I would rather have an interview by the one person in charge of the school. I did better that way. This time, it was okay. My experience in the psychiatric care facility came to bare. Experiences there impressed the mental health staff that were on the committee and helped me get the job. I finally arrived! This is the first job of all teaching jobs that I really wanted and I had the education, experience, and confidence to do it! Therefore, why not pray to get it?

I would start out on a pay scale with ten years experience, the equivalent of two master's degrees on the doctoral level of pay, and full county benefits with my family finally being blessed by all that, the way they deserved. No regular school district would do this for me, nor appreciate the knowledge and skill I brought to the job that the county would and not be afraid to pay me for it. I started in a class of junior high-aged. Earlier in my book, I labeled this age group as the most difficult to manage of the emotionally disturbed population. Because of their high energy and lack of impulse control, it increases volatility of their personalities. A good illustration of this happened during P.E to have a Multiple Subject Credential in California, which also covers Physical Education. My assistant and I joined a basketball game with our students. Toward the end of the game, as it was often a close game, the losers were poor losers and immediately had to fight. At that point, I had to break up a fight. Then we had to walk to the classroom. In that process, the fight would invariably start up again and I would have to break it up all over. This was all because somebody didn't like the results of the final score. Their tempers flare at the 'drop-of-a-hat' or quicker. It comes 'with the territory' in teaching this population. Impulse control becomes a major issue on getting this class under control. It was going to take time and patience.

A very strict behavior modification would be needed to fit this age group. Positive reinforcements that the students really want to work for are the key. The classroom rules have to be set and reiterated often, so the students are crystal clear about them. Fairly and consistently implementing the rules had to be imperative. In disciplining these students, I had to keep my emotions completely out of it. I absolutely could not show myself to be frustrated or angry. If I did, they will have considered themselves to have pushed my 'buttons' and it would perpetuate more negative behavior and would be seeing what other buttons they could 'push.'

Because of the nature of poor impulse control, it became important to 'not sweat the small stuff.' Let me explain. A teacher in regular education might not be able to handle annoying 'little' things that students may do in class that might be distracting to others. If the teacher allows it to 'get to him/her' it may become something that is overreacted to, wasting a lot of energy that could be used for something positive. Ignoring the behavior and finding a way to engage the student academically will cause the annoyance to dissipate without confronting it. Even more serious behaviors are ones we need to quickly and quietly squelch and direct everyone's attention back to academics with not more than a bump in the road. When you get to this point with a difficult to manage class, then you have good control of them! You ask me to 'get real.' Okay, if you have student that comes in completely upset from any number of things or you get a new student suddenly, then you may have to start all over to reinstall your system. This is part of teaching emotional disturbance.

Anything you learn from me here you are welcome to use of course. I designed a way to do PE, not everyone will be able to use it, but it worked well for me. As a teacher, or you may have an assistant that might be able to do this or even a PE teacher willing to teach your emotionally handicapped students, this may be of value to you.

This is two-handed-touch football. I had to design this to accommodate females; my school had boys and girls. I removed blocking from the line of scrimmage so a boy wouldn't hurt any girls. It became an all-passing game. Everyone is eligible to catch a pass. I chose to quarterback both teams. Because of the nature of the students and their handicapping conditions, it worked more smoothly this way. These students get frustrated fast and give up quickly! I was a quarterback when I was young so I could throw the ball to as many people as possible for more participation and the students were at least motivated to try. I divided the field into two or three parts for a way to earn a 'first down' or so many catches for a first down as agreed upon by the team captains. This became our PE, I tried to make it fun for all as much as I could. Girls felt good about contributing if they were fast, and the boys had a hard time catching them. My junior high students joined in bravely with high school aged students. I had to observe carefully that the older students didn't take advantage of the game situation and 'bully' the younger ones. I found myself needing to protect one student who seemed to have become a 'scapegoat' for the older bullies even though, for the most part, my PE project seemed to be working.

At this point I want to bring up an issue, and this student triggers that issue and one of the reasons I have a serious- problem with it. The State of California, back then, had started to pass laws affecting educators that would eventually force them to teach homosexuality as an alternative 'life style', as part of required curriculum in the state. It was not law yet, but that was the direction the movement was going.

This made me angry at different levels. First, it was going all the way from being a behavior that was against the law to being 'forced-down-the-throats' of the general public and now, our children! That was wrong! Now, I had a male student that 'triple-defined' this problem. He had been raped by his own father! The one man he should be able to trust in the whole world became a major factor in his emotional disturbance! It was my job to help put the pieces of his life back together and believe in him. He was soft-spoken, respectful, and a hard worker. The resilience in this young man was inspiring! When he participated in sports during PE, he wasn't the greatest athlete and was small in stature, but he played his heart out! I was proud to know him. I couldn't imagine being forced to teach this 'alternative life style' which is much more violent than you will ever hear on the six o'clock news.

Eventually, I moved up to a high school class. I had heard about grants being available to teachers. It was being offered by the Division Special Education at county headquarters. Teachers only need apply with amount and how it would be utilized. Of course, my application had to be accepted. I brought a bachelor's degree in Fine Arts-Music to my classroom; therefore I wanted to try to get equipment with which to teach music and drama. I put in for a video camera, a Roland synthesizer/keyboard; a music writing program, a small sound system, an amp., and a console piano and microphones.

Well, I got the grant including all these things! This teacher was a 'happy camper'.

You have heard of music 'taming the beast' going back to young David who played for King Saul, the first King of Israel. When dealing with students possessing the emotional disturbance, music can be a magic tool of therapeutic value and an amazing motivational incentive.

I developed my course of music appreciation for summer school. I taught some basic music fundamentals that could be used to play some songs on the piano. Classical vocabulary and genres were instilled in the students. Then I showed them videos of American folk music and their historical development. For instance, singing cowboy movies and TV shows did a lot to promote country western music. Appalachian Mountain folks had their own music. Negro spirituals or Black folk music was the basis for the development of Jazz. All this music was born in America.

As a response to the Beatles taking America by storm, American rock bands sprung up as a counter-revolution. These were all on videos to give students a taste of them. I also started teaching vocal music and teaching to read parts. So my music program was underway.

One of the great things about teaching keyboard skills is the value of incentives and motivation. Students from time to time that may have had a hard time focusing on their class work or were too easily drawn into negative behavior. If they are learning music skills on the keyboard, I gave them a goal to finish a certain amount of work for the incentive to practice on the keyboard with headphones. It worked like a charm, and if he/she was normally a behavior problem, suddenly the student was too busy to feed into negative behavior! My strategy for teaching disadvantaged youth music appreciation is about music fundamentals, reading music a little bit, as well as exposing them to all kinds of American folk music. America is rich in its folklore and music that many times gets neglected in regular education school curriculum. I had a student that made a profound impact on me for different reasons. He was a classic example of a student that needed music to help him focus. He started learning to play songs on the piano. It helped him on his schoolwork to get it done so he could get on the piano. His focus interruptions could have been negative input, or girls, but musical incentive minimized his distraction. It was amazing to me. Music had become so important to him that he was bold enough to ask the principal if he could play at graduation!

One of the most indelible memories I have of this student was that he was 'bi-polar.' There was a crisis developing from this fact and that he hadn't taken his medication he was supposed to take. It was a complicated situation in which to teach if your bipolar student hasn't taken meds, being effective as a teacher gets sabotaged at times by this situation.

Anger management is many times an issue with emotional disturbance. Each case has to be dealt with uniquely to the situation and the emotional makeup of the student. In this case, it involved my young music student. He was probably over six feet tall (taller than me). It was one of the most difficult anger outbursts I ever dealt with in my career! Luckily, one of my colleagues was a substitute teacher that was a former Beverly Hills Cop! He was big, probably 300lbs and I was over 240lbs. Even at that, he had to be trained in crisis intervention protocol that we had to use in this case.

This student completely 'blew-a-fuse' and we had to subdue him to keep him from hurting himself or someone else. It took all of our strength sustained for a long time to subdue him! It became the most dramatic story about a student that didn't take his meds!

In my situation at this school, parents or guardians were available to take students home the remainder of the day, or at least bring the meds they didn't take. Later, when I worked in probation camps, taking meds or not taking meds weren't so easy to deal with even though they had mental health workers there as well.

One more story about this student may be worth mentioning. I was so proud of his progress in our program that this incident really blindsided me personally, because no one could see it coming. Through the course of the day, some fellow students got a glimpse of a fairly large bladed knife in his backpack during moments when he opened it during class. He couldn't be allowed to go home on the school bus as the principal unraveled the situation. At this point, the deputy sheriff had to be involved. The student's story went like this; he had to walk across town the night before, through a dangerous part of the city, and had the knife for protection.

He forgot to take the knife out before he boarded the school bus in the morning. I believed his story. He was motivated to be in school and didn't want to miss. That meant a lot for me, but this was out of my hands. He was arrested for having that knife at school. The next school he would attend would be a probation camp school, locked up.

My next adventure in fine arts at this school had to do with teaching theatre. My approach in teaching theatre involved teaching all aspects of a production and involving as many students as possible. When I was working at the psychiatric care facility, I had made a friend of a young dramatist from 'off-Broadway' who had come out to Hollywood to produce and direct plays in his own small theater. I had shared with him ideas I had for a play. He liked my idea and wanted to meet over dinner to talk about ways to make my idea work. When we met in Beverly Hills for dinner, we stayed there until we had talked through all the things it needed to work.

The play was about a mayor of a medium-sized city facing some drug and gang-related problems. The mayor works with the city council and community leaders to find answers. One day, I checked my mailbox and found the play! My friend had sat down and wrote the play using all the things we had agreed upon!

My strategy as an educator for its use was to give adult roles to my students; either as parents or community leaders. They had to deal with issues of youth-related problems. I thought that somehow, psychologically, it was good for them to be on the other side of the issues and dramatizing them in a convincing fashion. The script was a little bit of a problem. It seemed to be quite crude in its language, too crude for school use. My students came up with the best replacements for the profane language. The really important parts of the play were exceptionally well written!

Then we built a rack to hold 'back-drops' for changing scenes. Students were used to help paint scenes. The play was going to be performed in the back corner of the classroom. We did not have a performing arts center or stage on which to perform.

We trained a stage manager and stagehands to change scenes. Part of the stage manager's job was to make sure the actors entered the stage at the right time and place.

It is a much greater challenge to teach here than at a regular education school. The nature of emotional disturbance is extremely 'touchy,' meaning, giving up at the drop of a hat; giving up on doing the play once a day; they need us to build them up and re-motivate them constantly; the dichotomy is that all kids are motivated to be actors at almost any age; and the emotional makeup of these students handicaps and sabotages their desire to act.

This makes preparing a performance extremely difficult! Teaching emotionally handicapped already requires more patience than you can imagine. To teach performing arts to these students is nearly an equivalent to insanity. Each day will give you more than you can handle. At least, you may think so often. I needed to have the attitude that I absolutely would not let the students sabotage the project, the play. Because we had boys and girls, I could not let their ever-shifting love focus or infatuations keep us from doing the play. Each day, I had to decide who couldn't focus for the day, work with the ones that could, and then come back to the others the next day! I had to take it one day at a time and not allow myself luxury of getting discouraged. If I did, it would be like shooting 'myself-in-the-foot.' It became important to have backup actors for most parts so they could take over if needed. The play about the mayor was performed. More parents and friends of the school attended this event than any other in the history of our school. One of the props was a round table about which the city council sat with the mayor. If the table stayed, it was transformed into a dining table so that through most of the play, the table was present. The value of this allowed actors to have a script in front of them flat on the table should they need prompting.

At one point, I discovered that I had a student almost eighteen years of age who did not know how to read! We obviously had to give him one on one attention everyday, but he was so excited about the play! We found a part for him. It wasn't a long part, but it was important. Several students relied on the script being there as a 'crutch' as you would have for a 'reading theatre.' But let me tell you, this guy had his part down 'cold!' It was memorized and stated in a convincing manner! I couldn't be more proud of him!

The special education units all across the county are always adjacent to a regular education facility. Even our school was next to a large high school. Occasionally, we would get a student that was more advanced in core subjects and closer to grade level skill. I remember a student that was able to integrate to a biology class next door. We became his support group to keep him encouraged. His success in that class was more important than most anything. We gave him extra time to study and helped him study for tests. All his others studies would fall in to place behind it.

As you recall, my version of PE football, we discovered a student with high-level football skills. We started jumping through all the 'hoops' to get him an opportunity to try out at a large high school football team. It worked, and I think it was the high school closest to his home that offered him an opportunity. He had skills and speed, all we cared about was for him to get a chance, and he did. As a staff, we proved we could do it, should we need to again.

We always offered summer school. That was a county-wide Division of Special Education practice. We had an interesting event that involved my youngest daughters at home and my students at school. At the last university where I studied music composition, they had a children's theater program in which they sometimes performed Broadway-type musical productions. This time, both of my daughters were involved. They were going to do *The Music Man*. My daughter came to me and said the professional barbershop quartet they had lined up to perform, quit the show. My daughter told the director I would do it because I performed it in college. The director asked to meet me and got my consent. The funny thing about it was that when I was in college, I performed the highest men's part in the quartet. This time, I would have to sing the lowest bass; I didn't have to learn the words, they were deep inside me. However, musically, I had to learn a whole new part.

My older of the two daughters involved wanted to qualify for the highest level dance team and she worked very hard to be designated as 'understudy' for the 'lead.' The lead, herself, was a college girl studying music and drama. My daughter was still in high school. My youngest daughter was an older elementary school student. This may be the only Broadway-type production all three of us would be in together.

Now, these productions were done for families and communities in the evenings. A few daytime performances were staged for schools to enjoy. When my boss found out about that, she wanted to bring students from my school and not tell them a teacher was going to be in the performance. It was a total surprise! I remember being out on stage and looking up into the blackened theater when I heard someone say, "Mr. Sills!"

As we worked with mental health department staff, we spent a significant amount of time together so that we were all on the 'same page' as problems and issues came up. Briefing and debriefing became important to the effectiveness of our staff and our ability to work together.

We were directly accountable to county-wide Division of Special Education. I got an opportunity to represent the north county area on a committee at county headquarters, devoted to program development for students with severe emotional disturbance. I felt honored to be on this county-wide committee and took the position seriously.

As the county provided educational programs for severe handicaps, more and more school districts were starting to take over the responsibility and provided their own programs. This was becoming problematic for county teachers, except when the school districts decided to give students continuity for their programs by keeping the county teachers. Otherwise, county teachers could look around the county for a position that might be open and their seniority would help them into opportunities. We had the only school of its kind in the county, at least public school. Word got back to us that our school was a favorite of the county Director of the Division of Special Education.

It was upsetting to hear that the high school district, where we were, wanted to take over our school. We didn't know why. Maybe they saw dollar signs. It took time to gather a staff and for them to learn to work together effectively.

It was their right to take over the school if they thought they were ready to run it. They did have to go through quite a bit of red tape to be able to take it. After all we had their students from all over the district.

In the past, school districts took over the education of severely handicapped students and it's harder than they expect and they are not prepared for it. The county has learned to run programs more economically efficient, so school districts have that to deal with, but it is their right to start and they have to start somewhere. Those of us on the staff, mental health workers, teachers, and paraeducators are only disappointed because after much hard work, we were becoming confident in each other and our program. We had received a principal who was up to the task, very good, and a highly qualified leader. This made the project even stronger. This was one of the best administrators I have ever had before or since! She saw the benefits of using my fine arts degree for the benefits of the students and was very supportive of my creativity.

12

To Lock-up!

It took time to be able to find another job within the county. Spending the time with younger students and those with mild to moderate handicaps helped me decide that for which I am suited. One, I need to be with high school-aged, and two, I am always drawn to the most severe or most difficult to manage. The county has a system of schools in conjunction with the probation department for incarcerated youth. I signed up for the open positions for which I was most interested.

After a while, I finally settled into a probation camp close to home, which I didn't really expect. We had twin camps, one for boys and one for girls. I started with the boys, feeling like I was a 'rookie' and needed experience in a whole new system, a set of all new expectations. I spent time learning how not to do things, and how I should have done things, like a 'rookie' in any field of occupation.

It was decided to make both camps 'girls.' That change seemed to be a good fit for me. I didn't know if it had anything to do with raising four daughters or not. Maybe it did.

To teach in camp, it was of great value to have my Multiple Subject K-12. For camp I would fit in anywhere. They may need me to teach any subject. Unfortunately, when I left working for the Division of Special Education, I also had to leave all the performing arts equipment behind that I had received from the grant. Another special education school got it and gave it a home. I started by teaching Language Arts and Reading. In adjusting to a new assignment, I had to get used to having temperaments of having all girls. They were 'whiney' and master manipulators. Most of them were also more conscientious in their schoolwork than the boys, generally. That was nice; it meant most of them were hard workers. To me, it meant as long as they are working hard, they are not distracting others. They have been in all kinds of trouble. They have been bank robbers, gun-runners, gang bangers, prostitutes, assaulter of teachers, and attempting murders

It may be important to know my philosophy for teaching in this situation. I did not go around asking what each student had 'done' to be sent to camp. I wanted to accept each student at face value and tune-in to their skills and lack thereof. I would then start believing in them and caring about them as a person so I could start building them 'up' to increase their confidence and self-esteem. I never got 'into' why they were in trouble unless it was to understand them, or for some reason they had a need to disclose it to me. Later on, I started a special education class and found it necessary to study some of their history more often as a need to help with their educational goals. I only wanted to consider it as a necessity.

It was helpful to have state approved Language Arts texts for tenth grade as it was devoted to American Literature. I appreciated this text as it had a wide variety of famous speeches, poems, plays, paintings, sermons, and fictional entrees from all different historical settings in the history of the United States. It was a rich resource to teach these students. This was especially valuable because of having students that are many times deprived of American culture. There are different reasons. One is that they may not have been in school much because of running-the-streets. Prior educators or school systems may not have taught this important homegrown American literature. It doesn't matter too much why. It gave me an open door, an opportunity to enrich their educational experience.

During this time of teaching Language Arts, I had to be certified to teach English for language learners. I did have a majority of Hispanic students so I could use the practical value of the certificate, as part of the requirements. I wrote a forty-page research paper. Within that research, I found something that was profound to me personally, maybe because a big part of my heart is an artist. The research that grabbed my attention had to do with the findings of psychologists on the East Coast. They believed there were a higher percentage of gifted and talented students among the incarcerated population, as opposed to regular education students. This became a new mission, to find a few of these students and create an opportunity for them to shine. Bachelor's degree was in Fine Arts-Music, as well as fort-five units of graduate school in music. This gave me ample background for the challenge. As we were considering budgets for our school, we got an opportunity to apply for federal funds as individual teachers. The county gave us guidelines to help us be successful in our inquiry. That was appreciated. My thrust would be in the direction of music and drama. My philosophy of teaching theatre, I mentioned earlier, was to teach students every aspect of drama production, involving as many students as possible.

This time, my funds would be used to teach music and drama after school. I also put in for funds to spend on building materials to use to build drama flats for scene backgrounds. My design of these was such they could be used over and over. They were put together with nuts and bolts so they could be broken down and stored if necessary. The music part was to put in for keyboards/synthesizers and headphones so students could learn skills and have incentives for their regular work. A transferring colleague donated a small piano to my classroom. We were thankful and adopted it.

The actual performance rehearsals were after school. I had learned that this way, I could work with the students that really wanted to do it. It was too difficult to do it with a regularly scheduled class. The students that didn't really want to do this became distractions and made it difficult to focus and teach others.

13

Camp Theatre

After school, I could weed out the students that really didn't want to do this. After that, I could accomplish much more. The next part of this was materials. I had accumulated music, famous songs well known from Disney movies, and Stevie Wonder songs. From these, I carefully picked songs that I could re-arrange in parts so I could teach the girls to sing soprano and alto parts in harmony.

As far as drama, I had to write them a play to perform. Plays for all girls that are meaningful to them, and educational as well, don't grow 'on trees.' I got the concept of creating a play that transports these girls from the street and crime, to the world of being adults and businesswomen.

All of the women would be employed by the same corporation, and decided to go out to dinner together after work, thus the title of the the play was *The Dinner*. They would all be dressed in suits or nice clothes. What do I have them talk about? Current events that are issues, relationships with men, and being mothers; I injected my own wisdom, and history of women in the United States. This way, they get healthy ideas about being women in this modern day world of grown-ups, and then turn around and dramatize it. Logistically, smaller table groups were spread across the stage. Each table had their topics to talk about, one table at a time. They were addressing individuals in other groups didn't happen until closer to the end of the play.

I had a contact with someone in the costume business in Hollywood. She graciously donated costumes for my 'project.' The students were 'made up,' hair fixed, and dressed up for women in the business world. We built flats for the background and painted them. For the students that didn't have parts memorized, the scripts were lying flat in front of them. A little idea that I carried over from my past production, each actor in this play sat in front of a round dinner table making this possible. There are some interesting stories behind my next production that I want to visit. I needed to come up with a contrasting story line and allow for more dramatic talent to shine and develop characters more than in the last one. Being in Southern California puts anyone in 'earthquake country.' How could I make a meaningful plot on that fact? I posed this question, how could an earthquake change people's behavior? In life, people naturally have conflicts between personalities and in family relationships. How would these relationships and conflicts be changed if suddenly, there was an earthquake? Would they be changed for the positive? I was going to set up three groups of women, related in different ways. One would include a hard to handle teen being raised by her grandmother, and an aunt that stopped by occasionally to check on them. Another situation included two college-aged sisters with their single mother. The third scenario involved a teen living with her single mom and grandmother.

It was fun creating these characters as they developed tensions or annoying relationships setting up an interesting place for a natural disaster to happen, and creatively spin the premise that people change when disaster hits. As each group is a family group, will attitudes change when the earthquake happens? That should make a good question to answer as the drama unfolds.

The first production, *The Dinner* was involved in building flats, backgrounds for the play which the students painted. This time we upgraded the design of the flats. We attached heavy duty wheels to the bottom of the flats. Why? This enables us to turn the flat around to change the scene. A different scene would be painted on the back.

It was important to have rehearsal after school so that I had the students who really wanted to do this. The play also took place around a kitchen table in each of three different scenes. The practical aspect of this was to be able to lay a script flat for the parts that weren't memorized.

We had to plan for waking up on the day of the play and be missing a character for the performance. There were things that could happen suddenly that I had no control over. One, probation could take students out of camp on transportation in the morning. Because of this, we needed to prepare students to 'cover' more than one part and rehearse them. Another way students could miss the performance would be if they get in a fight. If they got in a fight, they would be put in solitary confinement automatically; and if it were a major actor, somebody had to be ready to cover the part. Juggling the parts around the last minute was a possibility. I had to plan for not unlike managing a baseball team.

There were simple scene changes that took place as well as planning on modifying them for after the 'earthquake.' Stage hands had to be trained for scene changes. The most invaluable student was my stage manager. The stage manager knew everything that needed to be done and who needed to do it. I made one big mistake with this production, something not obvious. The morning of my play my stage manager got drawn into a fight! She was never in trouble and the most conscientious student I knew. You would think someone deliberately sabotaged our play. My mistake was that I planned for everyone to be 'covered' except the stage manager! I didn't have anyone trained to do her job. Once she was drawn into a fight, she was locked up in solitary confinement and I was stuck without her!

A day or two before the performance, during our rehearsal, we had an earthquake and it felt just the way I described it in the play! That was amazing, as if inspiring our play! As the play unfolded, the characters put aside their annoyances and focused on each other and their safety. Thus, people and their attitudes did change in the wake of the 'quake.' They refocused on 'what' was really important in life. Family and safety became most important and the realization that it was great just be alive!

I called my play *Quake!*

14

Camp Music

In starting from 'scratch' to teach music at the camp was going to require some creativity. It was going to be important to teach them songs that were 'catchy' tunes. It was important to find Mariah Carey songs that they knew. There was an uplifting song that I taught wherever I went, *For Once in My Life* as recorded by Stevie Wonder. This is so 'catchy' the students would walk around singing it. That blessed my heart to hear. I was always looking for lyrics that were upbuilding in some way. Mariah Carey's *Hero* became one of the those. Not only did it inspire a student to 'belt-out' a solo from it, the rest of the girls joined in on most of the song.

I needed a song in which I could teach the girls to sing parts, harmonizing with each other. I picked the duet, *A Whole New World*, which was from a Disney movie *Aladdin*. The song was a duet by Aladdin and Jasmine. I loaded the piano accompaniment in the computer to play so I could get the computer to play the piano, in order for me to direct the song with my hands. Once in a while, I would play. The students worked hard to harmonize, and they liked *A Whole New World*, so that became a motivating factor for them to learn.

As a colleague was teaching fashion design, she gave me a standing invitation to perform at a fashion show during intermission.

When we did sing at the fashion show, I pulled out some more Stevie Wonder songs like *Isn't She Lovely*.

When we did sing, it was a time when we were being reviewed for our school to be accredited with Western Schools and Colleges. We were having a reception for the Accreditation Committee. The principal, my boss, wanted the girls to sing at the reception. We sung only once, but she was so happy with their singing, she added them to the activities around the reception. We did it and I was proud of them as well!

In and around this activity, I had a student that had been creating some impressive sounds and songs on the synthesizer. I showed her how to make recordings on the synthesizer. I hooked up speakers to simplify it so people could hear what she had created as a prelude to the girls' singing.

I had twenty singers. Within the last couple days, I had had more girls begging me to let them sing. Without them rehearsing with us, I couldn't let them sing! That was motivational for all of us nevertheless.

It was an advantage to be able to offer performing arts to our students and nice for the consideration of accreditation. As long as my administrator supported my fine arts, she left funds in the budget for me to teach after school. This was a glowing gesture of confidence!

15

A Special Mission

I was called into the principal's office. She said that we had staff members with experience in special education, but I was the only one on our faculty that was fully credentialed for what she needed. She needed someone to start a special education class. It would keep us from being out of compliance with state law to offer a Special Day Class that would service students from both camps. If I volunteered for this assignment, it would save my boss from going to all the trouble of hiring someone. I had to consider that I had a master's degree in Special Education including learning handicapped, emotional handicapped, and emotional disturbance. These students are why I got this education. So I needed to go for this assignment! I had to move to a class next door at the other camp. I was used to receiving a new class every two hours during the day. Now, a Special Day Class would mean I would keep my students all day for every period and every subject as before.

Considering one of my major tasks would be modifying extreme behaviors, it was actually helpful to have the students all day. Somehow, if you had problems with a student early in the day, and gave time for the situation to mellow out, many times I was able to motivate students to get back to work and even catch up work from the morning.

It was to my advantage that because of my class being than a regular camp class, and camp classes were already limited themselves because of the nature of incarcerated youth. Once I got started, because of the extraordinary energy required for dealing with the most difficult to manage behaviors in camp, I couldn't have taught fine arts after school. My energy was spent.

My boss brought by a higher up administrator, Director of Juvenile Court Schools for the entire county. As she brought him into my classroom she said, "This is the most patient man in the whole world, and that's why he is here." I didn't expect her to say that. I had to accept it with grace and as a compliment. He was familiar to me and had been in my class over at the other camp.

An important thing to establish, first off, was behavior modifications, strict rules and incentives for following them. Being fair and consistent is all important; something the students can 'count on.' I was going to get students that were emotionally disturbed and that were with bipolar disorder. We did have the help of mental health department. In my situation, I was better off to reach out to those workers either to help understand my students that were particularly needy of getting suggestions for strategy which was also helpful. I did reach out to them from time to time and found it invaluable.

A number of probation camps use a point system for behaviors throughout the day and throughout the week, honoring the students at the top or most improved. It was going to be more important to me if probation followed through with their point system and even offered them a 'store' once a week where they could 'spend' their good behavior. It was important for any special education kids because I could then design my behavior modification to tie into what they have established.

If probation did not have a consistent point system in operation, then it became imperative to design my own for each hour, each day, and each week. For me, the most points for the week earned Student of the Week. Good Grams I made for daily, usually weekly for best in a particular subject or improved work habits, or attitude. These are printed and placed in the students' hands as they left the classroom. Once in a while, a student needed to build on very short term success. They either didn't have any success in school for a long time, or have been out running the streets and not been in school at all, or had a disorder that was making it hard to focus for very long. At any rate, finding something important that would be suitable for positive reinforcement was very important. The student may not be capable of finishing an assignment, so the teacher may have to set a goal like to finish a certain amount in thirty minutes. Let the student play a music keyboard with headphones, on computer, or listen to music for so many minutes, great incentives.

Another way to help a student who was having a hard time with their probation officer might need a daily Good Gram that they could take to the PO. Their goal might be to have one really good day in school. Hopefully, they would like the feel of it, and follow it with another good day. Many times the 'feel' of success perpetuates good behavior and hard work.

One of the major challenges lies in motivation. One day, as I was coming to work and walking to my classroom, one of my students was having an extreme big girl 'tantrum' before a couple of probation officers. She was extremely disrespectful towards them. They seemed at a loss to know how to respond to her. My secretary told me she was the most difficult minor for anyone to deal with in camp and she would be in my class! Usually, if someone is describing a student, my attitude inside was 'let me have a shot at them.' This is the first child I remember that needed my attention quite badly.

I am sure it took a lot of patience. I believe in demanding respect which the probation officers weren't getting. At the same time, I want to do things that earn respect as well. Part of the plan means giving the student respect even though they might not deserve it. Treating them politely even though they may not seem worthy.

This particular girl has a different side to her story that I remember more readily than anything else. Recall "music tames the beast?" This fits her in a different way. There was a certain kind of music that I approved of and happened to be a kind she liked. It brought a miraculous change in this young woman! I turned on the music, she asked for her school assignments and got to work. Before our eye, the worst became the best, and the most focused on school work.

It is important for me to inject something of an issue here. Some teachers and administrators would not have a problem with what I just described, given the nature of my students. Some would have a problem. The topic here is music to work by. This again is a therapeutic function of music as described much earlier in the book to help self-abusers.

There are times when it is expedient to direct teach and other times when there needs to be quiet seat work. I absolutely could not allow rap or hip hop, styles that are perpetuating and glorifying life of the street; crimes, drugs, sex, and violence from whence my students came.

All this goes toward motivation. Music can have a mellowing affect on our classroom and even more valuable for my students that have emotional handicaps. These students have the shortest tempers and short attention spans. A little music works magic on these temperaments.

What you can do depends on the day and the class and how they respond. If they have a problem with my choice of music or get to complaining or whining about the music my simple solution is that it goes off immediately!

It was an advantage to have had crisis intervention training many times over and be trained to be a trainer. I could catch a conflict before it got 'carried away.' I remembered a girl that entered the classroom provoking a gang-related fight before she even sat down! She was immediately removed with the help of probation officers! I also remember before she left me, that she became a motivated, hard-working student! She was out quickly, what I wasn't going to tolerate and my parameters were going to be strict, so she might as well settle down and study. She found out I cared about her and didn't hold grudges from one day to the next. In fact, I didn't allow emotion or anger to be a part of my discipline. I have talked about this before. Anger doesn't motivate kids.

Each day was a new day, to be positive, and expect the best of my students. Most of the time when students have been in fairly serious trouble, they can calm down and be more cooperative as well as respectful. That kind of respect has been earned. I was able to demand respect in not allowing any kind of fight provocation and then turn around with kindness and caring, and help the student with their basic skills in the classroom

Another strategy important for these kinds of students, incarcerated or emotionally disturbed was to not allow myself to be pulled into a 'power struggle.' (This is also good to use at home). It can start as an argument with a student. If you are the teacher or parent, and already decided what you want to happen, you have to 'stick-by-your-guns,' and stop the conversation. Don't get sucked into a power struggle. If they wear you out and you finally give in, you lost! And you gave them power they didn't need to have! They won't stop there, they will be wielding power again as long as you allow them. At the very beginning of the argument, you have to be able to 'put on the skids.' You have to be able to say, "this is my decision, conversation over." Don't argue with them. Don't talk about it.

Academically, a special education classroom like this had interesting challenges. If I gave everyone subjects according to age, I would have five or six different levels going at the same time. If I had taught everybody the science they were suppose to be studying, it might be four different subjects and same for social studies or civics. By looking at the students records and what subjects they should be taking, it sometimes made things more complicated.

One of my problems was giving them 'grade-level' work when they didn't have the skills to 'handle-it.' When I made vocabulary lists, it usually included words from different academic disciplines such as, Social Studies, English and Math. When students were too low, I gave them a modified spelling list picking out the easier words, but they had to learn what the harder 'words' meaning and how they were used. That is, they were learning the grade level words even though they were not 'up-to' spelling them. They were tested on their meaning. Sometimes, I made a crossword puzzle of vocabulary to test vocabulary usage ability.

Teaching math in this class was a little 'tricky.' Students may need to take algebra or geometry and be weak in basic skills. I tried to set it up so that I took time to work on basic skills and additional time to work on algebra and geometry.

The only kind of camp classroom that had a paraeducator to assist the teacher was a special education class. When it came to math, it was a big advantage to have some help. I usually had a wide variety of skills with which to deal. For instance, it is easier to learn basic algebraic manipulations if you know your multiplication tables. Depending on the students, I may have them learning both. There are basics of geometric calculations that are common to algebra as well. These allowed me to do direct teaching to the entire class and involve all students, especially if they needed to learn

If I had one student more advanced than anyone else, I would get them started where they needed to be, explain how they are going to do it and hope I had a paraeducator that could help as I return to the rest of the class.

With the help of a teacher's meeting which discussed new strategies and approaches, as part of my assignment, I created a math game. This was math bingo. I had to make it beneficial to my entire class with a wide range of math skills. This, I had to do on my computer. Answers to the problems had to be on the bingo cards. Each card different with only some answers that were common. That idea was to plan problems to fit the answers. Each problem would be written on the blackboard (or whiteboard). Some problems would be fundamental math knowledge like measurements; some problems that students did through the rest of the week. For this to work and keep the pace of the process moving along, students were supposed to speak up with the answer until someone came up with the right answer. Once in a while, we stopped to explain how we got the answer, for the kids that maybe didn't know. This made more of a learning experience than it might be. I let as many people get a 'bingo' as possible, so we played 'til we 'blacked out.' We always played right before morning break and gave them a nutritious snack for getting 'bingo.' This activity was motivating and a fun way to review the week on Fridays, especially if not done every week. Any teacher reading this is welcome to use my ideas and adapt them to your own classroom.

A different kind of methodology swept through our camps, and as teachers we were taught how to use it. Primarily, it was more and more direct teaching which was modeled for us, ways of engaging the students more actively and checking for understanding very often. An outgrowth of this more effective teaching enabled camps to be teaching the same chapter of each subject as the next camp. This made it possible for students to be relocated anywhere in the county and not really miss school assignments or chapters of learning.

Algebra was on chapter ten all over the county; US History was on chapter twelve all over the county. I learned a lot about teaching more directly and more effectively. It just so happens teaching special needs became more complicated and more impossible! I had to teach five different levels of social studies and by the time I taught it all directly, my school day would be over, having covered one subject matter. If it were necessary to abide by the new format for instruction, it was going to be quite impossible.

16

PBL Comes to Our School

Project Based Learning was going to revolutionize the way we taught and learned at our school. It deserves mentioning in this book for the positive changes and positive results. It became extremely noteworthy for special needs students; at least from my perspective.

In an age of technology and standards for learning, it is hard to imagine momentarily putting standards aside. At that time, state standards seemed to be overworked and all and because of this, teachers began to teach in the direction of teaching to tests rather than subject matter, and the maturity of students' problem solving skills and critical thinking. It might be important to mention California has a greater number of students to educate than any other state. Because of the wide variety of cultures and languages, it should increase the bias against the standardized tests and lower the overall test scores across the state. To compare it to the rest of the country becomes an unfair assessment.

Caucasians have become a minority to Hispanic population with English as a second language group over all standardized test scores. It is my opinion that standardized tests shouldn't be held in such high esteem as a priority for assessing students' skills and teachers' effectiveness. It should only be a limited tool. My view is that it became such when politicians got involved in what should be important. I think politicians should leave education to educators. Education is so much more than a score on an objective test, which only tells what the students don't know, not what they know. There is so much to a student nowadays; the student's emotional make-up, self-esteem, moral support or lack thereof, and varied adversity in their life that may have affected their learning and many times a factor. Students come to school having had to adjust to parental divorce, broken families, and without moral support from home for their education. They have come from a home of drug abuse, molestation, or domestic violence.

A single parent or grandparents may be trying to manage being the adult and too many jobs, this makes the child to run the streets or just simply fend for themselves without adult supervision. This sets them up to be recruited by a street gang, or at least without the support at home needed for healthy development as a student.

These are all adversities for the child to fight through, and add to the burden of a caring teacher who has to be everything to that child. Thank goodness there are programs for children who come to school hungry. A compassionate teacher may be able to lighten the load of the baggage children bring to school, so that school becomes the most anticipated part of the child's life. In that case he or she will be highly motivated even if the skills need to be caught up in different areas. These things can't be measured by a test.

PBL was new to camp schools and the incarcerated youth, but it was not new to the county. We got to be first as a camp school. It was going to be interesting, as I was now teaching a Special Day Class. What kinds of responses will I get from my special students in this program? That was the question. I was about to engage in the adventure to find out.

The first project would be different than each of the ones to follow, but we had to start somewhere. This was an experiment in education for these kind of students. This doesn't mean it hadn't been done before somewhere, just not with me and not in this county.

As a staff we needed extra time to together. We had to brainstorm so we could write the 'script' as we go, since this was new to all of us and no curriculum to follow.

What we decided for the first project included researching occupations of interest. This was interesting to me because it got our students thinking about legitimate ways to make money. Most of my students had been making money illegally, by stealing, robbing, prostituting, running guns, running drugs, or robbing banks. It was interesting to find out how this subject matter might get them to 'dream-a-little.'

We didn't have but staff computers in my classroom, we had two. My paraeducator was good at helping with research even though we only had two computers. I found that the US Department of Labor had a large website that was very detailed on many occupations and comprehensive to the training needed, the salaries to be expected, and demand for workers in that field. As the girls chose occupations they really want to research, we printed out a stack of information for them to study, and on which to take notes. If they enjoyed doing hair, they may have chosen cosmetology.

Part of the requirements was that each student had to also document places they could go for training; beauty colleges or even the government program. Job Core, where they offered cosmetology as a program and provided a place to stay, if the student met the requirements for admission.

Another part of the requirements was for the students to prepare a power point presentation of their findings. They had to write an original script to go with it. A short essay was required, at least one page, describing ways this project had been important to the student personally.

Because we were handicapped by not having student computers in our classrooms, the only way to get the 'power point' part of the project done was to give students time on staff computers. They had to have the script handwritten so that all they needed to do was type it in.

Because several of the girls had chosen cosmetology for their project, I decided to 'dream' up a large math problem in which each student would be put into the perspective of the owner of a beauty shop franchise. The objective would be to calculate the earnings of the beauty shop for a month.

I got a haircut with the owner of a beauty shop franchise. While I was there, I asked her all kinds of questions, enough to help me create the problem and make it realistic. The students acting as the owner/ manager had to create a work schedule for the employees including themselves and days off for all. They are given the prices for all different hairdos and haircuts for men and women. Every week, they had to schedule a variety of cuts and perms and not all the most expensive sittings. Everyone is limited to the same chairs and same number of workers. They had to add up monthly expenditures and include $3,000 franchise payment. Figure in fair workers' salaries. Then for the month, compute how much your shop has made (or you) after all that. It should take three or four days to complete this problem. One or two periods per day, doing it carefully until finished.

At this point I am not teaching music or drama because of the demands of Special Day Class in this setting (camp school). I am thrust into a program that requires a great deal of teaching creatively and I was just getting my feet wet. From that time on, my creative juices would have to get flowing in a variety of ways. It is important to describe some of those ways and the evolution of the processes as we developed PBL in our school.

One of the first rather dramatic observations I made, had to do with motivation. In dealing with special education students and especially emotionally disturbed, motivation can be a major issue to be worked on everyday and all day at a variety of different levels. Some of these students are hard workers from day one. Overall, girls have been more conscientious than boys. Some of the students come into class with their own agenda. They have a predetermined plan to what they are going to do in class and what they are not going to do. One way we used to describe it was that 'they are running their own program.'

This particular time, I had at least one of those in my class. She was quite noteworthy at the time. She was the most difficult minor to deal with for the probation officers in camp. In class, she was a challenge for me because of her predetermined agenda and would only be motivated to do the school work the way she wanted. To get her to do what I wanted her to do when I wanted her to do it, I had to out 'con' as in the 'con artist.' Every day was new in trying to figure out how to motivate her and getting her to be compliant.

This student was in my class when we started PBL for the first project. She had chosen cosmetology. She was as dramatic a story as I have to tell about the transformation PBL made in behavior and motivation! May I remind you, she was the number one most difficult child for the camp probation staff. She was always doing her own thing.

As she started her project, she totally changed! She came to school excited and motivated 110% to get started on the project! When she got to the stage of doing the power point, she was greeting me at the door enthusiastically, and wanting to be the first student on my computer and her project! This was an awesome transformation of motivation and defiant behavior!

My next most dramatic happening with this girl went like this, the first and only time I ever got a visit from the County Superintendent of Schools happened after we had been working on this project for a while and each student had a three-ring notebook full of research materials and work from determinations made by students. My student, the subject of this story, had her desk near my desk and mine was near the entrance to the classroom. Any high ranking administrator that I recall from the County Office of Education, said a quick 'hello' to me and immediately focused on the children and turned to them. The County Superintendent was no different.

The first minor for him to meet was the closest! Even though she had worked very hard on the project and greatly minimized her negative behavior, she wasn't very cooperative at first. He had no idea he was talking to the number one most difficult kid in camp. It was an amazing experience I won't soon forget, to observe him matching wits with her and he was up to the task. It took time, but he finally had a breakthrough. He had discovered that she had written her one page essay. She lit up like a light bulb and decided she had something he might appreciate, finally. She pulled it out and he was very impressed which made her quite proud. She probably had no idea who he was or even what a County Superintendent was. She had met her match in the wits department!

The Superintendent met with us teachers later in the day and shared that he was impressed by an underlying enthusiasm and motivation by our students for the change in our program. He said he was beginning to observe the learning experience the students had to go deeper in understanding than they may have learned in a textbook. He also shared that our school had become a priority of his, across a vast county of two million learners. He promised to support our program in any way he could, and keep close tabs on how we were doing. I believe we actually started receiving technology upgrades for the classroom including a smart board and computers for students, whether it was the superintendent's doing or not. We did have an aggressive and creative administrator that could account for it as well.

One of our next projects included a study of the Holocaust. A math project calculated how many bodies could be crammed into a railroad car/container similar to a 'cattle' car. Students also designed a 'dollhouse' to fit the description of the hideaway in Anne Frank's Diary where she and her family hid from the Nazis. Students studied the Holocaust from a greater number of perspectives than I had ever seen in standard curriculum.

At the end of a unit in school when all the projects are ready for display, we had an open house for visitors from the county office or other schools, family and friends. An agenda was chosen for each class and a hostess (student) or ambassador became somewhat of an emcee and narrator to each group of visitors. One rule was that the teachers didn't say anything about the students' projects, the students did.

When there was a number of different projects around the classroom on display that were earth science projects, the hostess took the guests around the room and allowed students to explain about their projects if needed. The earth science projects included a study of Mount St. Helen's and aftermath studies and updates. Another was a model built of the CO^2 cycle in the earth. As we learned about the BP oil spill all, different aspects of it were studied and the recovery effort. Alternative energies were studied including auto fuel made from sugar cane in Brazil, and also biofuel being created in University of California, Berkeley Lab invested by BP.

One of the student's experiments showed how difficult it was to deal with oil that had come into water and onto sand of a shoreline. It really opened the eyes of the students working on it. As projects were delved into like this, the learning experience that is more practical and deeper than the standard textbook/lecture format was evident. This was born out by visitors who were educators and administrators.

No matter what the main thrust of the projects were, most of the time, teachers created math to relate to the projects. Knowing the skills that were needed for the math portion of the projects we got our math, algebra, and geometry texts and drilled students on specific skills needed. We also documented specific state standards by number that were required from the text.

One of the last projects that I was a part of included visitors walking away from my class, they were asking and wondering if my class was the 'advanced class.' How exciting was that for my kids? Our guests were never told we were a special education class! For one thing, a student can be emotionally disturbed and also be very bright and have a high IQ. When it came to having a hostess for our class, she many times had high energy, enthusiasm, and very articulate in which case people enjoyed them and their presentation! Why throw cold water on all that by saying this is a "special education class?"

One of my colleagues that was primarily a math teacher and I collaborated to create a project for stock market investment. Each student was given an imaginary $10,000 to invest. The students all invested in the same five companies chosen by the teachers. The students made the decision of how much to invest in each company. They created charts, graphs, and portfolios. They documented the performance of their stocks. At the end of the quarter for the 'open house,' we determined which student earned the most money on their investments. They learned to make several kinds of graphs and the state standards were documented to show what math skills were learned for the project. It was fun and the students were proud to show visitors their portfolios. They even designed their own covers for their portfolios. They were very tastefully done.

Through all this time of launching into PBL, as a staff, we observed much less conflicts between teachers and students and students on students, most of this because students were motivated and engaged in learning. To look around my class and see them busy most of the time, you wouldn't believe them to be special education And as far as the dilemma of having students eighth to twelfth grades and wrestling with how to make sure everybody is studying what they are suppose to be studying;, Project Based Learning was 'heaven sent' for the deeper comprehension in learning that was observed, and the dramatic decrease in extreme behaviors!

Before entering into my final chapter, I wish to gratefully acknowledge the probation staff who were kind, patient, and mentoring me when I needed it most! Our partnership was invaluable!

As a preface to the final chapter, I describe two of the most dramatic tales I have to tell you and how I dealt with them, and then I skip back into an autobiographical mode to end the book. Keep it in mind should the ending be offensive to you.

17

The Gospel According to George Washington

In the nation's capitol is a prayer room with a stain glass window of George Washington kneeling in prayer, which has also been a painting. George Washington and what he had done with the Continental Army in the Revolutionary War was nothing short of miraculous! He took teenagers and humble farmers from thirteen colonies and defeated the greatest army and navy in the world from Great Britain! Washington was already a military genius, but was constantly in prayer over his men. Contrary to what you may have heard about our founding fathers, Washington was a man of God and a man of prayer! Why am telling you all of this? It will make sense a little later.

Up until the summer of 2012 I was teaching high school in a probation camp for Los Angeles County. I had been in schools where I taught classes of all boys; but the last several years I taught all girls. These students were locked up for stealing cars, robbing banks, pushing drugs, prostitution, 'gang-banging', assaulting teachers, attempted murder, or just violating probation. Before I retired, this job had gotten even tougher because I had started a special day class (special education). Because I got students that were severely emotionally disturbed, or they had behavior disorders, bi-polar and other mental health problems it meant that I had the worst behaved students in the whole camp all in my classroom and they had to stay there all day for all subjects. This was a stressful teaching job with a capital 'S'.

One of the most dramatic stories I could tell you from camp, happened in the afternoon. Because of what happened that day, I couldn't tell you what I had planned to teach! My students filed into class and sat down for roll call. Then one of the girls, barely fifteen years old, started coming unglued like she was about to have a nervous-breakdown! She was absolutely and completely 'scared to death!' I had never seen anyone so frightened! The other students seemed supportive and wanted to know what it was all about; so we put our seats in a circle that included her!

I knew that a number of my girls came from a scary world of life and death; but I had never seen anyone so scared! We were all very still as she told her story: she had been kidnapped, abused, and forced into prostitution. She was not even fifteen years old yet. Her mother did not know what happened to her. To her mom she had fallen off the edge of the earth! She was no where to be found. Why was she so scared now? She was locked up and in a fairly safe place.

The FBI had been to visit her. They wanted her to consider testifying against the guy that kidnapped her and forced her to prostitute herself. She was scared to death of ever seeing him again, even guarded by U.S. Marshalls in a courtroom! She was too scared of the very thought! She didn't think she could do it! She told us that he was the Devil in a human body. She knew "he had killed other girls." She was way too frightened to consider the request.

I was a public school teacher, but I needed to bring God into this traumatic situation. I had a favorite saying of George Washington in my pocket calendar. I read it to her as the rest of the class waited for some significant leadership from me.

> "May we never fail to consider the omnipo-
> tence of our God, who alone is able to protect."
> (George Washington)

I asked her if she knew what 'omnipotence' meant. No? All powerful: the God who created the universe, hung the stars in the heavens, flung the planets into orbit. This God alone is able to protect… You. I could see George Washington praying for the protection of his men often, throughout the war.

My student eventually calmed down. The other students and I pledged ourselves to supporting her and helping her gain courage, confidence, and faith to do this thing. Go to court! That first week she went to chapel - 'church' service for the incarcerated minors. We had two or three months to help her strengthen her courage before she saw the Feds again!

Thanks to these powerful words of George Washington, she built up faith, courage, and confidence by the time she needed them! She turned around so completely before she left camp, I chose her to be my Student of the Month. With the help of George Washington, we brought God into the equation, and she built her faith in God through it.

The second student I would tell you about, came to my class weighted down with a heavy burden. She was very quiet, very polite, and respectful. Some students I would get were extremely disrespectful. For them to be defiant, refuse to do what they were told or curse me up one side and down the other – many teachers would not last a day in my classroom. I had my ways of dealing with those behaviors, but it took time and patience.

This time, the student was quite respectful, and seemed to want to busy herself with schoolwork. At some point I detected the heavy load she was carrying. She finally told me, knowing she couldn't hide it any longer. Her boyfriend had been killed in a gang related shooting! But this was different. She claimed that she and her boyfriend were not gang-related! So what was different?

They were at a funeral in which there was gang-related gun-fire. Her boyfriend suddenly ran and dove in front of the gunman's target! He saved the life of a friend, but it cost him his own life! That story immediately takes me to the words of Jesus in John Chapter 15:13 – "Greater love has no one than this, than to lay down one's life for his friends." This story had a deep impact on me. The student in my class didn't want to leave my side. She wanted to be in a desk near my teacher's desk. She chose to help me in any way she could. She passed out papers and books. She did the work of a T.A. with the greatest attitude, grateful that she got to be in my class. She was a real blessing to my class of short tempers and disrespect.

Recently, I had watched a movie about Navy Seals thwarting a terrorist plot against the USA. Real Navy Seals were used for the story, "Act of Valor". Near the end of the story as the terrorist plot was being foiled, one of the Seals dove on an explosive device to save the lives of his fellow Seals. That took me back to my college years during the Viet Nam War. One of our football playing buddies had become a U.S. Marine. He came by the Nazarene college I was attending to play some sand lot football down by the girls' dorm. If he was on the other team you had to keep a forearm up or he would hurt you. He was so strong!

He had come by to say good-bye before he boarded the plane to Viet Nam. He played football with his friends, then left. The guys that took him to the airport said he turned to them and said "I don't think I'll be back."

A couple years later news came into the Senior men's dorm that he had been killed. The movie was make believe but this was real! We were told that he dove on a 'live' grenade to save the lives of fellow Marines.

He was in harm's way for his friends that were home and free to go to college. I took it personally, what he had done in service to his Country, which included me. This sacrifice hit close to my heart!

People can be given over to a list of sins found in Romans Chapter 1. For me to end on a positive note that I want to do, I need to take a couple minutes and talk about sin. The recent election in the State of Washington including passing the same-sex marriage issue as law. Romans 1:24 says "Therefore God also gave them up to uncleanness, In the lusts of their hearts, to dishonor their bodies among themselves, who exchanged the truth of God for the lie, and worshipped and served. The creature rather than the Creator, who is blessed forever, Amen.

"For this reason God gave them up to vile passions. For even their women exchanged the natural use for what is against nature. Likewise also the men, leaving the natural use of the woman, burned in their lust for one another, men with men committing what is shameful, and receiving in themselves the penalty of their error which was due.

"And even as they did not like to retain God in their knowledge God gave them over to a debased mind, to do those things which are Not fitting; being filled with all unrighteousness, sexual immorality, Wickedness, covetousness, maliciousness; full of envy, murder, strife, Deceit, evil-mindedness; they are whisperers, back biters, haters of God, violent, proud, boasters, inventors of evil things, disobedient to parents, undiscerning, untrustworthy, unloving, unforgiving, unmerciful; who, knowing the righteous judgment of God, that those that practice such things are deserving of death, not only do the same but also approve of those who practice them." Romans 6:23 says "The wages of sin is death." I got sick of the woman making TV commercials in favor of 'gay marriage'. She always said "We are all God's children..." In God's Word it's different. John 1: 12 – says "But as many as received Him (Jesus), to them He gave the right to become the children of God, to those who believe in His name: who was born, not of blood, nor of the will of the flesh, nor of the will of man, but of God."

Now I want all of you to close your eyes and imagine there is about A seven foot long altar down at the front of the church sanctuary. Imagine you are placed on the altar to be sacrificed next. Suddenly, a voice loudly Says "Wait! Wait! Your debt has been paid! You will not have to pay for Your own sins with death! Someone has taken your place! He was the perfect sacrifice, because he was tempted in every way that we are but did not sin!

God wants you to rise up and be a living sacrifice serving Him all your days. (You may open your eyes.) Now let me take you to the kind loving words of Jesus from John Chapter 15: "As the Father loved me, I also have loved you; abide in my love. If you keep my commandments, you will abide in my love, just as I have kept my Father's commandments and abide in His love.

"These things I have spoken to you, that my joy may remain in you and that your joy may be full. This is my commandment that you love one another as I have loved you. Greater love has no one than this, than to lay down one's life for his friends. You are my friends if you do whatever I command you. No longer do I call you servants, for a servant does not know what his master is doing; but I have called you friends, for all things that I heard from my Father I have made known to you.

By receiving Jesus as the Son of God we have the right to become children of God. We have to be given that right! Jesus laid down His life for us - His friends. He made an example of the Greatest Love! We have gone all the way from talking about the protection of the God of George Washington – to discovering the 'greatest love' in Jesus terms and the fact that Jesus wants us to be more than servants… He wants us to be friends!

The difference between religions and Christianity should be this: "relationship." This adventure of life is a friendship with the Son of God that wants to bring us into the family of God.

About the Author

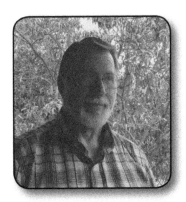

After working with youth and children for forty-seven years, Gary David Sills is retired from teaching in the classroom. His days are now filled with sharing his storehouse of knowledge with others, spoiling his fourteen grandchildren and volunteering in several areas at his local church. He is busy writing church music and dramas, which has always been a dream of his to pursue.

CPSIA information can be obtained
at www.ICGtesting.com
Printed in the USA
LVHW042029031119
636213LV00001B/24/P